THE NATURAL WAY
OF HEALING

WOMEN'S HEALTH

The Natural Medicine Collective

Dr. Brian Fradet, D.C.
(Coordinating Panelist, Chiropractic)
Dr. William Bergman, M.D. *(Homeopathy)*
Brian Clement *(Nutrition)*
Elaine Retholtz, L.Ac. *(Acupuncture)*
Dr. James Lawrence Thomas, Ph.D. *(Psychology)*
Dr. Maurice H. Werness, Jr., N.D. *(Naturopathy)*

with
Rebecca Papas

A DELL BOOK

PRODUCED BY THE PHILIP LIEF GROUP, INC.

Published by
Dell Publishing
a division of
Bantam Doubleday Dell Publishing Group, Inc.
1540 Broadway
New York, New York 10036

Note to the Reader:

This book is not for the purpose of self-diagnosis or self-treatment, and should be used only in conjunction with the advice of your personal doctor. Readers should consult an appropriate medical professional in all matters relating to their health.

Produced by The Philip Lief Group, Inc., 6 West 20th Street, New York, New York

Copyright © 1995 by The Philip Lief Group, Inc.

ISBN: 0-440-21661-3

Printed in the United States of America

Published simultaneously in Canada

April 1995

10 9 8 7 6 5 4 3 2 1

RAD

WORK WITH THE BODY'S
INHERENT ABILITY TO HEAL . . .
AND NATURAL THERAPIES FOR . . .

ENDOMETRIOSIS AND BENIGN UTERINE
(FIBROID) LUMPS

Suppressed feelings of anxiety are a hidden factor in these conditions. **Psychotherapy** and **hypnosis** can help you discover the root of this emotional imbalance; and **affirmations** will reinforce the mind-body connection to healing.

PMS—ESPECIALLY FATIGUE, IRRITABILITY, CRAMPS

Get immediate alleviation of symptoms from the **essential oils of aromatherapy** used in a bath treatment of rosemary, lavender, chamomile, and lemon. This wonderful stress break is soothing, restorative, and a true pain reliever!

MORNING SICKNESS

Sometimes it may seem as if *nothing* can be done for this common problem of the first trimester, unless you take potentially dangerous drugs. Not true! **Acupressure** is a gentle, safe treatment, using points on the arm and calf to give you relief!

CANCER PREVENTION

Enhancing the immune system and stopping the damage of free radicals are aims of **nutritional therapy,** and you'll find the facts on specific diets that some claim have produced "miracle cures."

PLUS

PELVIC AND YEAST INFECTIONS
BENIGN BREAST LUMPS • PREGNANCY • MENOPAUSE
OSTEOPOROSIS AND OSTEOARTHRITIS

THE DELL NATURAL MEDICINE LIBRARY

Health and Healing the Natural Way

**LOOK FOR THESE OTHER TITLES IN
THE DELL NATURAL MEDICINE LIBRARY:**

*Stress, Anxiety, and Depression
Chronic Pain
Asthma and Allergies*

Contents

THE NATURAL WAY
OF HEALING

WOMEN'S
HEALTH

Introduction

Women today are juggling many roles. They are managers and psychologists, physicians and athletes. Many are mothers, too, so they race from boardroom to nursery, changing diapers as often as athletic shoes. While women-on-the-go seem to have a limitless energy supply for accomplishing goals, they must be careful to avoid neglecting their needs by overworking, eating poorly, depriving themselves of sleep, and not allowing time for the pursuit of interests outside of work.

All of these can lead you to imbalance, throwing your body and mind out of whack and making you vulnerable to illness. The notion of keeping balance in life is not new—sages have espoused this wisdom since ancient times. Maintaining balance is also a primary tenet of natural medicine.

Natural medicine is a system of health care that recognizes the body's inherent ability to heal. This healing ability is enhanced by promoting balance across the many facets of your life—the spiritual, emotional, physical, and psychological components. In recent years, natural medicine has surged in popularity because of its individualized and preventive approach. While conventional medicine employs standard treatment based on patterns of disease, natural medicine recognizes that each person experiences illness differently, and shapes treatment according to your unique needs. Perhaps most important, natural therapies are inherently preventive—by incorporating natural therapies in your daily routine, you can correct an imbalance *before* it turns into illness. While we have been conditioned to think of treatment only when we become ill, natural medicine offers therapies that are gentle enough to become part of our lives so that we are building health day by day. Natural therapies like exercise, nutrition, meditation, and yoga, when practiced regularly, can improve a woman's physical and emotional health, lowering her susceptibility to disease. These therapies, in essence, are preventive as well as curative.

Because self-care is integral to its approach, natural medicine encourages a woman to garner as much knowledge as she can about her health. This volume of the Dell Natural Medicine Library is intended to lay the groundwork for self-care by providing you with enough knowledge to begin self-applications.

By reading this book, you will learn:

- How psychotherapy can be effective in relieving anxieties that can underlie conditions like endometriosis and uterine lumps.

- Which healing foods can minimize health concerns such as menstrual pain, minor vaginal infections, and nausea.

- How to apply acupressure therapy to relieve minor energy imbalances that can lead to conditions from cystitis to morning sickness.

- When to seek chiropractic treatment to improve muscoskeletal strength and alleviate a variety of health concerns from osteoarthritis to menstrual problems.

- How to make herbal preparations to treat a range of ailments, including the hormonal fluctuations of menopause and the side effects of conventional cancer treatment.

- When in-depth acupuncture treatment can be helpful in relieving energy imbalance before it manifests in health problems such as vaginitis and breast lumps.
- How to employ simple relaxation techniques like breathing and meditation to reduce your susceptibility to illnesses such as osteoporosis and cancer.
- Which homeopathic remedies can be effective in alleviating common complaints of pregnancy, menopause, and many other conditions.
- How to exercise to reduce health risks and minimize the pain and discomfort of conditions like osteoarthritis and menstrual problems.

This book is organized so as to first give you an overview of natural medicine and of therapies that are at the forefront of this system of health care. In the first two chapters, you will learn how natural medicine differs from conventional medicine in its concept of illness and its methods of diagnosis and treatment. You will also learn how to find a natural medicine practitioner. In subsequent chapters, you will learn how to apply therapies, including Oriental medicine, homeopathy, chiropractic, psychotherapy, herbs, exercise, and many more to specific conditions. A brief overview of these chapters is given below.

"Maintaining Health" describes therapeutic techniques for fulfilling the most important tenet of natural medicine—prevention. Besides explaining self-care techniques for relieving emotional, spiritual, and physical imbalance, this chapter offers suggestions for daily and weekly preventive regimens.

"Menstrual Problems" unveils a wide range of natural therapies for treating one of the most common and vexing women's health concerns. Addressing realms such as the psychological, nutritional, and metabolic aspects of this condition, this chapter extensively explores the underlying causes of menstrual problems and offers many suitable remedies.

"Pelvic Infections and Benign Gynecological Concerns" examines a wave of pressing women's health conditions—cystitis, vaginitis, endometriosis, breast and uterine lumps—their origins and influences, and presents an array of approaches to treatment. Besides investigating nutritional and psychological factors, this chapter surveys important emotional influences as well.

"Pregnancy" takes a look at this multifaceted natural process and its impact on all aspects of a woman's life, and provides knowledge for complementing conventional prenatal care. In addition to covering important nutritional and physiological concerns, this chapter provides techniques for enhancing delivery and for preventing the physical and emotional strains associated with childbearing.

"Menopause" surveys the many aspects of this important passage with an emphasis on the whole person and recommends many therapeutic techniques for preventing and relieving discomforts. Not only does this chapter address symptomatic relief during menopause, but it also elucidates health concerns that can develop in later years, offering preventive strategies.

"Breast and Female Reproductive Cancers" illuminates the many forms of natural therapy available to cancer patients for supplementing conventional cancer treatment. Besides describing techniques for ameliorating symptoms of cancer and the side effects of treatment, this chapter highlights preventive strategies.

"Bone Health" explores two predominant diseases among women, osteoporosis and osteoarthritis, and explains a variety of therapeutic applications. Not only does this chapter cover methods of symptomatic relief, but it also elucidates metabolic approaches for preventing or slowing the progression of disease.

In the chapters ahead, you will learn that one of the most important advantages of natural medicine is its recognition of the healing power of not just the body, but the mind as well. From meditation to yoga, biofeedback to hypnosis, imagery to psychotherapy, these therapies utilize the mind's remarkable ability to promote your health. This tenet, which has been integral to natural medicine for centuries, is at last beginning to be validated by Western research.

New, ground-breaking research, in fact, has transformed the concept of the "mind." Once thought to be only the brain, the mind is now believed to have a presence throughout the entire body because the cells which carry emotion have been found throughout the body, not just in the brain. Cells that carry emotion are also found in the body's immune system, offering evidence that our emotions and the immune system are inextricably linked. Some researchers question whether the receptors, or links, for these emotion-carrying cells that are found in the immune system *compete* with virus receptors for entry. In other words, they suspect that some of our emotions may play a direct role in preventing certain illnesses. Another study that seems to back up this mind-body link showed that women with metastatic breast cancer who participated in group therapy lived twice as long after diagnosis as women who did not participate in such therapy. Group therapy had provided positive emotional benefits to participants that nonparticipants had presumably not received.

Given this evidence of the mind's powerful influence, it is no wonder that natural healers, who typically acknowledge and nurture a patient's emotional needs, reap wonderful results. Not only do natural healers increase a patient's trust, they also may be augmenting a patient's healing potential!

Despite the differences between conventional and natural medicine, or perhaps because of them, the optimal approach to health care may be a combination of the two schools of thought. Natural medicine assesses the symptoms of illness as a sign of a deeper instability or imbalance within a person, and tries to restore physical and mental harmony. Conventional, or allopathic, medicine focuses mainly on the "course" of disease and its treatment. An integrated approach aims to produce a health care with a full knowledge of the person and the illness, not just the illness, one that is less harsh and invasive, one that is individual, yet based on collective experience. Natural medicine provides a gentle and long-term approach to maintaining health, while allopathic medicine is essential in treating serious, life-threatening emergencies and some acute illnesses. If we combine the strengths of natural and allopathic therapies, we could produce a powerful medicine of the future.

An example of the powerful healing effect of integrating natural and allopathic medicine can be found in the case of a girl ill with a dangerous outbreak of lupus (lupus is a chronic condition that affects many parts of the body including the kidneys). A team of experts lead by pediatrician Karen Olness at Case Western Reserve University needed to administer doses of a potent drug to get the disease under control. However, because the drug suppresses the immune system and could have put the girl in danger of developing other illnesses, practitioners could not continue administering high doses of the drug to the patient. Thus, they paired the patient's doses of the drug with the taste of cod-liver oil and the smell of a fragrant rose perfume. While practitioners cut back significantly on the dosage of the drug, they continued to administer the cod-liver oil taste and rose smell without the drug. The powerful sense of smell and taste effectively convinced the mind and body that it was receiving the same dosages of the curative drug. Remarkably, lupus symptoms did not reappear.

You will learn more about the healing abilities of natural medicine in the journey ahead. Our goal is to help you to take charge of your health, restore balance in your life, and maintain health without the use of drugs or surgery. Because you will experience varying success rates with different therapies, experimenting is recommended to enhance your overall knowledge. You'll find that some therapies listed in forthcoming chapters, like acupuncture and chiropractic, require the services of a skilled professional, while other treatments, like massage, can produce great results with just the help of an enthusiastic amateur. Herbs, acupressure, meditation, yoga, and many more applications can be self-applied in your own home. Initially, you may want to complement knowledge of self-care by setting up a consultation with a professional or by taking a class. However, even without that supplement, you will learn enough from this book to greatly enhance your knowledge of how to obtain and maintain good health. Please note that the information in this book is not intended to replace your traditional medical care. It should be used in conjunction with the advice of your physician. You should always consult an appropriate health professional before undertaking any treatment or making any medical-related decisions.

CHAPTER ONE

What Is Natural Medicine?

Acid rain . . . the disappearing ozone layer . . . smog . . . radiation . . . contaminated well water . . . It has become evident, from media reports as well as from personal experiences, that our increasing knowledge and technology can both help to advance society as well as wreak havoc on our lives. In a similar way, as the science of medicine has become more technical and has made great strides in treating many illnesses, it also has become more and more manipulative of and invasive to the human body. Unnecessary surgeries, excessive medication, life-support mechanisms . . . all of these alter the natural processes of health and illness, life and death. One cannot deny the value of surgery and medication in treating certain ailments and diseases, but it seems that we often lose sight of the body's power and ability, with the proper care and nurturing, to heal itself.

This notion of healing oneself is at the root of natural medicine philosophy. As more people witness the harmful effects of technology and the overuse of conventional modern medicine, they are turning to alternatives that are less invasive and disruptive of the body's natural processes. The new "health-consciousness craze" of the 1990s is all around us. People are striving to eat the right foods and maintain their proper weight; more people have made exercise a regular part of their daily routine; and some have discovered the benefits of relaxation and meditation, two elements that are particularly vital in our fast-paced, hectic lives.

You might grant that diet, exercise, and stress reduction are all well and good, yet doubt that they are a sufficient means of curing specific illnesses. How can riding the Lifecycle for twenty minutes three times a week possibly help chronic acid indigestion? The missing link is the mind: Proper care of your body helps create a healthy mind, and a balanced mind leads to a healthy body. They are interrelated; some believe they are one and the same. As a society, we are skeptical—we like to have things proven through testing and experimentation, and we like to see the facts. The brain and neurological system can be viewed as the physical embodiment of the mind, and this is true to the extent that scientists and doctors can measure and test these vital organs. The mind, however, is more than a mass of nerves, hormones, and electrical impulses. It represents an invisible, intangible, yet extremely powerful energy that, unfortunately, we often are too quick to dismiss.

Throughout history the mind has been viewed as something that must be mastered and controlled, otherwise one might "lose one's mind" or "go out of one's mind." An inability to control one's mind signified personal weakness to many people. It is useful, however, to think of the mind not as something to be controlled lest one go mad, but as energy to be harnessed and used to restore and maintain overall health. Indeed, this is the underlying philosophy of the practice of natural medicine.

Vis medicatrix naturae—the healing power of nature— this is the premise of natural medicine, which involves the use of an array of noninvasive, natural therapies to help restore balance to the body and thus help the system to heal itself. These therapies, which will be discussed individually in Chapter Two, include Oriental medicine, homeopathy, hydrotherapy, botanical medicine, physical medicine, psychotherapy, biofeedback, and nutrition. Natural medicine discourages the use of treatments that weaken the body's innate ability to heal itself, and although a person sometimes requires more than natural remedies, the natural medicine practitioner will always try to use the least invasive treatment possible.

Natural medicine functions from a holistic point of view; that is, your whole being is treated, rather than simply the part of your body that is sick. Natural medicine practitioners will take into consideration not only your obvious and immediate symptoms, but lifestyle, psychological factors, and other physical imbalances that may be present. They believe that illness affects the whole person—physically, emotionally, and mentally—and that imbalances within and among these three spheres will cause a person to exhibit symptoms of sickness. Natural medicine requires you to become involved in your own healing and to claim responsibility for your own health. Doctors have long been considered teachers of a certain kind, and natural medicine practitioners continue the tradition of educating their patients to become more aware of their own bodies, emotions, and minds and to help the self-healing process along.

Natural medicine strives for a balance between mind and body. If appropriate and necessary, various therapies can be used concurrently, or they can be used to supplement standard medical treatment if the case warrants it. The fact is that no one remedy or therapy—whether it is conventional or alternative—can work for everyone all of the time. The key is to explore your options and use the treatment that is most successful in treating your overall health and well-being.

Natural therapies are gaining popularity as people increasingly realize that conventional medicine cannot always offer all the answers or cures. According to a study published in the *New England Journal of Medicine* in January 1993, approximately one-third of all Americans used alternative medicine therapies in 1990, including relaxation techniques, massage, macrobiotic diets, spiritual healing, self-help groups, biofeedback, acupuncture, hypnosis, chiropractic, herbal medicine, and homeopathy. Patients spent $10.3 billion on alternative health care in 1990, and 90 percent of the treatments were sought by patients without the advice or suggestion of their regular physician.

The mainstream health-care industry, likewise, is changing to keep up with the growing demand for alternative medicine. The National Institutes of Health, at the urging of Congress, established an Office for the Study of Unconventional Medicine Practices and an Office of Alternative Medicine in 1992. Some conventional physicians have incorporated natural medicine philosophy and technique into their own practices. Insurance companies such as the American Western Life Insurance Company of California, the Mutual of Omaha Insurance Company, Blue Cross of Washington and Alaska, and the New Jersey–based Prudential have extended coverage to include natural therapies. Clearly, natural medicine is becoming more popular as patients seek alternative treatments to those offered in Western medicine.

DIFFERENCES BETWEEN CONVENTIONAL AND ALTERNATIVE MEDICINE

Standard, conventional, or orthodox medicine, also called *allopathy*, defines health as the absence of disease. This definition is based on a negative. In contrast, holistic medicine concurs with the definition of health used by the World Health Organization (WHO), which posits that it is a state of complete physical, mental, and social well-being.

The allopathic and holistic definitions of health differ greatly in regard to the diagnosis and treatment of illness. People who use conventional medicine usually do not seek treatment until they become ill; there is little emphasis on preventive treatment. Holistic medicine, in contrast, focuses on preventing illness and maintaining health. The best illustration of this approach is the fact that ancient Chinese doctors were paid only when their patients were healthy, not if they became ill.

Natural medicine, which follows a holistic approach, views illness and disease as an imbalance of the mind and body that is expressed on the physical, emotional, and mental levels of a person. Although allopathy does recognize that many physical symptoms have mental components (for example, emotional stress might promote an ulcer or chronic headaches), its approach is generally to suppress the symptoms, both physical and psychological. Natural medicine assesses the symptoms as a sign or reflection of a deeper instability within the person, and it tries to restore the physical and mental harmony that will then alleviate the symptoms.

Except for cases of severe physical trauma, most illness derives from a level of susceptibility that varies in different people. For instance, some people seem to catch every cold and flu virus that goes around, while others can go for years without so much as a sniffle or a cough. The level of susceptibility reflects the deepest state of one's being. Bacteria and germs, as well as carcinogens, allergens, and other toxins, are agents of illness waiting to prey on a susceptible host. These stimuli alone do not cause illness, but rather induce specific symptoms in susceptible persons. Certain bacteria are known to be associated with certain diseases, and there are bacteria living within our bodies all of the time. Hence, if bacteria were the cause of illness, we would probably be sick all of the time. Instead, illness occurs when an imbalance in the body allows the bacteria to reproduce uncontrollably. Natural medicine usually views this uncontrolled growth as a manifestation of disease, not a cause of it. Natural medicine practitioners believe that preventive medicine, or therapies designed to maintain and enhance health, can reduce people's susceptibility and therefore the frequency with which they become ill.

Because of the fundamental differences in the way that allopathic and alternative physicians define and view health and illness, they also assess and treat their patients in very different ways. Alternative practitioners believe that people can use the power and positive energy of their minds to defend themselves against disease. Symptoms, therefore, are not caused by illness, but reflect the body's best attempt to heal itself. Since allopathic doctors believe that symptoms are caused by disease, they also believe that alleviating the symptoms will foster cure. In contrast, the natural medicine practitioner will claim that suppressing symptoms fails to address the underlying cause of illness and, in fact, can drive the illness deeper into the body, causing more profound symptoms to develop.

For example, if a child has a fever, an allopathic doctor might prescribe acetaminophen. Although this can help to bring the fever down, it is not curing the illness, which must run its course. An alternative practitioner, on the other hand, would consider the fever to be an indication that the body is fighting the illness. A high temperature makes the body unsuitable for bacteria to grow, and so it is the body's natural defense against the infection. Of course, an excessively high fever can be dangerous and should be treated so as to reduce it.

The difference between allopathic and natural treatments also can be seen in relation to the common cold. An allopathic doctor might suggest using an antihistamine to dry up a runny nose. However, natural medicine believes that the flow of mucus, and indeed all bodily secretions, is significant to the healing process, as it rids the body of toxic substances. If you are the kind of person who likes the quick remedy—that magic syrup or pill—and does not want to endure the discomforts of illness in the recovery process, you will have to assess whether natural medicine is appropriate for you. All of the alternative therapies discussed in this book require that your mind be open to their philosophies and that you become an active participant in your own recovery and health promotion.

In allopathy, diagnostic testing is vital in order for the doctor to name and categorize the disease and to treat it. Often these tests are done routinely, sometimes for the purpose of protecting the doctor rather than actually to help the patient. Some diagnostic tests, such as excessive X rays, or the use of powerful drugs can even cause sickness, referred to as iatrogenic illness, meaning "doctor-caused."

Although modern holistic doctors might use some standard diagnostic tests, they are more concerned with the individual's life circumstances. When you visit an alternative practitioner for the first time, he or she will consult at length with you, or "take the case," as it is called. During this initial visit, which can last more than an hour, the doctor will interview you, making notes about your verbal and nonverbal communication. The practitioner will be careful not to compare you with another patient, as each individual is unique. The doctor will record his or her observations of you as well as your complaints and concerns and will most likely ask questions to better individualize the case. If you are seeking help for an acute illness, the doctor probably will focus on symptoms and feelings that have changed since you became ill. If you are complaining of a chronic ailment, the doctor will want to know as much as possible about your life and history. Conventional diagnostic testing can be useful in certain cases, but the alternative doctor's practice of "taking the case" allows him or her to get at the deeper source of your problem, rather than just treating your symptoms.

Natural medicine operates on Hippocrates' theory of *primum non nocere*, or "first do no harm." The goal is to treat illness with noninvasive, harmless remedies that invoke the body's innate healing powers. Natural medicine involves a comprehensive view of health, illness, treatment, and cure that meets the need of each individual person and helps to restore and maintain balance of the body and mind.

In some cases, natural treatment can suffice to cure an illness, but other times allopathic treatments are required. If this is the case, alternative treatments can still be used to enhance the effectiveness of allopathic medicine, providing maximum healing for the individual. Healthy individuals also can pursue natural medicine regimens to maintain and enhance their physical, emotional, and mental well-being.

HISTORY OF NATURAL MEDICINE IN THE WEST

The word *naturopathy* was not used until the late nineteenth century, although its philosophy originated with Hippocrates, whose school of medicine existed around 400 B.C. Earlier, people believed that disease was caused by supernatural powers. Hippocrates devised the theory that everything natural had a rational basis and that the causes of disease could be found in natural elements, such as air, water, or food. He also believed in *vis medicatrix naturae*, or the healing power of nature, and that the body had its own ability to heal itself.

The years from 1780 to 1850 marked the Age of Heroic Medicine. During this time, "heroic" treatments, such as bleeding, intestinal purgings, and blistering of the skin, were used to cure patients of their ills. These treatments were painful and harmful, and they often made patients worse, or even induced death. It was believed that bleeding, accomplished by lancing a vein or using leeches, removed impurities from the body. Intestinal purgings were performed by using mercuric chloride, which today we know causes severe metal poisoning; vomiting was induced by using other poisonous substances. The Age of Heroic Medicine was male-dominated and elitist, excluding women and nonconventional doctors. Some physicians who opposed heroic medicine practiced alternatives such as herbalism.

In 1810, a German doctor named Samuel Hahnemann (1755–1843) became disenchanted with the standard medicine of his day and began the practice of homeopathy. *Homeopathy* is derived from two Greek roots meaning "similar" and "disease, suffering." It is a philosophy of health and cure that is based on the principle that like cures like. That is, natural substances that produce particular symptoms in a healthy person can cure a sick person with those same symptoms.

Hahnemann did not actually originate the philosophy that like cures like; Hippocrates and others also had explored this concept previously. However, he did develop the theory into a viable alternative medical practice, homeopathy, which is discussed in greater detail in Chapter Two.

When Hahnemann died at the age of eighty-eight in 1843, he had many followers in Europe. The first homeopathic doctor came to the United States in 1828. In 1836, the Hahnemann Medical College opened in Philadelphia, and the first national medical society, the American Institute of Homeopathy, was established in 1844. As people began to react against heroic medical practices and politics, the Popular Health Movement was formed. It called for the repeal of all medical licensing laws, which was achieved by the end of the 1840s. This allowed physicians to practice whatever form of medicine they believed in. It was in this atmosphere that homeopathy flourished in the United States and set the stage for other alternative medicines, such as naturopathy, to take root.

Realizing that they were losing their foothold, the allopaths organized the American Medical Association (AMA) in 1846. While attacking homeopathy, they tried to give allopathy a more positive definition by claiming the word was based on German roots meaning "all therapies." Allopathy thus began to allow that a variety of remedies could be effective in treating a disease. The AMA required state medical societies to expel homeopaths and alternative healers, and in the 1860s, charges often were brought against allopaths who associated with these doctors. Allopaths began to wrest control of city hospitals and boards of health, and they succeeded in reestablishing licensing laws in all states. As the Popular Health Movement dissolved, alternative healers virtually were driven out of practice and denied any political influence.

By the 1880s, the homeopathic movement was being destroyed not only by the AMA but by its own internal philosophical divisions. Two groups of homeopaths emerged: those who were pure homeopaths, called Hahnemannians, and a larger, more modern group that included allopathic practices in their work and that wanted to work with allopathic doctors rather than against them.

Dr. John Scheel of New York City coined the word *naturopathy* in 1895 to connote "nature cure." The earliest forms of natural treatments and preventions included good hygiene and hydrotherapy. Naturopathy began to be pursued in full force in the United States in 1902 by Benedict Lust, who had emigrated from Germany in 1892. He had grown dissatisfied with conventional medicine and was intrigued by the European health spas, especially their treatment involving water cures and fasts. By the end of the nineteenth century, water cure was recognized as a vital healing therapy and referred to by the term *hydrotherapy*.

Lust intended to practice and teach hydrotherapy in the United States. Soon, however, his followers broadened their practices and healing philosophy to include an array of modalities, such as nutritional therapy, herbal medicine, homeopathy, spinal manipulation, exercise, hydrotherapy, electrotherapy, and stress management. Lust believed that in order to achieve good health, people should eliminate excessive consumption of toxic substances (such as caffeine, drugs, and alcohol), exercise, strive for a good mental attitude, and amend their lifestyles to include natural remedies such as fasting, proper diet, hydrotherapy, mud baths, chiropractic, and the like. He opened the American School of Naturopathy in New York City, which graduated its first class in 1902.

Natural medicine became very popular in the United States in the early twentieth century until the mid-1930s. At that point, conventional medicine again began to rise to prominence and popularity because of several factors. First, chemical and drug industries, which benefit more economically from allopathic than natural medicine, financially supported foundations that subsidized conventional medical schools. Second, orthodox medicine began to use less harmful treatments, and advances in health-care technology, particularly in surgery, convinced the public that conventional medicine was superior to natural medicine. The orthodox medical arena again began passing legislation that either limited or prohibited alternative health-care systems from flourishing.

Within the past two decades, since the 1970s, natural medicine has begun to take hold again. Realizing that allopathic medicine may not have all of the answers or cures for their ills, people are seeking alternative treatments. As people begin to recognize the devastating contaminating effects of some technology on air, water, and food, they are also beginning to take action against such harmful practices. Finally, as the connection between the mind and body becomes ever more apparent, people are willing to make major lifestyle changes in order to protect and maintain their sense of physical and emotional balance. This is what natural medicine is all about and it is why more and more people are realizing the long-term benefits of alternative medical treatments.

LOCATING A NATURAL MEDICINE PRACTITIONER

One of the best ways to find a good alternative practitioner is to be referred by one of his or her patients, though you might not be fortunate enough to find one in this way. At the end of this book is a list of Natural Medicine Resources. Contact the listed organizations. Often they can make referrals to practitioners in your area, or they may have membership directories available.

When consulting a practitioner, interview him or her to learn as much as you can about the person and his or her practice. As a result of the interview, you will feel more comfortable seeking help from this person if you decide to do so, and that level of trust and comfort will facilitate a beneficial outcome for your treatment. The American Holistic Medical Association can send you a publication, *How to Choose a Holistic Health Practitioner*. The organization's address is listed in the Natural Medicine Resources section. Following are some questions to ask a practitioner you interview:

- What schools did you attend and what is the extent of your training?
- What licenses or certificates do you hold?
- How long have you been in practice?
- What are your diagnostic and treatment procedures?
- What are the fees involved? What is the length of treatment or number of sessions proposed?
- Have you written any articles or books? (If so, they may be worth reading.)

CHAPTER TWO

Natural Therapies:
An Overview

ORIENTAL MEDICINE

Oriental medicine defines health not as an absence of disease, as in Western medicine, but as a total state of well-being. It requires that the body be free from physical pain, but also encompasses the totality of the individual's thoughts, emotions, and beliefs. Health, in Eastern philosophy, is a state of mind and a way of life. Illness results from going against the natural laws of Heaven and Earth.

Oriental medicine began at least three thousand years ago, and has developed progressively as a science since approximately A.D. 200. It continues to flourish in the Eastern countries today, and many aspects of Oriental medicine are beginning to gain popularity as alternative treatments in the West. Oriental medicine involves several healing therapies, including acupuncture, herbs, nutrition, exercise (such as tai chi chuan and other martial arts), massage, and manipulation.

Taoism, Confucianism, and Buddhism are the underlying philosophies of Chinese medicine. According to Taoism, health reflects a harmony in Heaven, which is achieved through the balance of external and internal forces. A unity exists within the diversity of nature—a universal energy that exists in all things. This energy, called *chi,* is very difficult to describe. It has been explained as matter on the verge of becoming energy, while at the same time it is also energy on the verge of becoming matter. Everything in the universe is a result of the never-ending condensation of *chi* into matter and dispersion of *chi* into energy. In terms of Chinese medicine, *chi* needs to be understood in two ways. First, it nourishes the mind and body and has been described as the life force. Second, *chi* is produced by and indicates the function of the various *zang/fu,* or "spheres of function." *Zang/fu* refers not to a specific organ, such as the liver, but to the totality of body functions associated with the liver. Stomach *chi,* therefore, refers to various stomach functions, such as the transportation of food essences. The Chinese believe that *chi* flows throughout the human body. Health reflects a free flow of *chi,* but if the energy is imbalanced—if there is a blockage, an excess, or a deficiency of *chi* in specific body parts or organs—disease and illness occur.

Taoism also recognizes two opposite yet complementary qualities to all aspects of physical being. The philosophy derives from the notion that the universe was originally a ball of *chi* surrounded by chaos. When this mass of energy finally settled, it divided into the two opposing yet complementary qualities called *yin* and *yang.* Yin represents qualities that are negative, contractive, dark, small, of the right side, interior, of the nature of Earth. Yang, in contrast, is positive, expansive, light, big, of the left side, surface, of the nature of Heaven. All objects, animals, peoples, times, and places are a combination of yin and yang. It is believed that people are born with perfect yin and yang balance that is later thrown off kilter. Chinese doctors designate certain organs as being either of yin or yang qualities, and so are the foods and medicinal herbs that would be used to treat ailments of these organs.

Practitioners of Chinese medicine and philosophers believe in a dynamic cycle of evolution known as the five-element theory. All things are classified according to the five elements of wood, fire, earth, metal, and water. The body's organs are also characterized by the five elements; for example, the spleen and stomach are of the earth, and the lung and large intestine are of metal. These five elements are in a state of constant change and interact with one another. Doctors believe that organs affect other organs according to the elements. For instance, wood generates fire; therefore, the activity of the liver, which is characterized by wood, generates the activity of the heart, which is a fire organ. The relationships between the elements show doctors the direction in which *chi* flows within the body.

Just as the Chinese views about health differ from Western notions, so do their ideas about human anatomy. Chinese doctors identify twelve organs, or the *zang/fu*, which do not correspond directly to organs as we know them. Remember that *zang/fu* refers not to a specific organ, but to all of the body functions associated with that organ. This way of looking at the body probably evolved because ancient Chinese tradition prohibited the opening of corpses. Therefore, rather than developing a more detailed, concrete knowledge of anatomy, scientists and doctors focused on body functions instead of specific organs. The result is a more holistic understanding of function that embraces physical, mental, and emotional aspects.

Chinese medicine requires that the flow of *chi* in the body be influenced or moved, either by the practitioner or by the patient, so as to restore its balance. The flow of *chi* can be impeded by poor nutrition; lack of exercise; mental stress; fatigue; bad posture and breathing; pollution; physical growths such as tumors; or trauma, including those that result in scar tissue. A deficiency in *chi* can cause fatigue, depression, and various physical ailments. Excess *chi* might be responsible for hypertension, migraine headaches, or some types of arthritis. If the natural flow of *chi* through the body is altered in any way, a host of ailments could occur.

Chi flows through the body in fourteen pathways called meridians. The geography of the human body, as viewed by Eastern doctors, is based on these pathways as well as the *zang/fu* (organs) and bowels, and is very different from Western concepts of anatomy and physiology. Twelve of the meridians pass through a major organ and are linked to other meridians, so that all body parts have access to *chi*.

Practitioners of Oriental medicine examine and diagnose their patients in a way that is quite different from the quick, routine examinations and consultations patients in the West are accustomed to. There is careful questioning and observation of the patient, as well as monitoring of the patient's pulse. This is not pulse-checking as we know it, however. Rather, it is a fine art of detecting several layers of pulses in order to determine which body spheres are suffering. The doctor will take a pulse using the first three fingers of his or her hand, checking the patient's wrists with both light and firm pressure. The doctor will also identify pulses under each finger at both pressure levels—a total of six pulses for each wrist. Each pulse correlates with a specific body function sphere.

Acupuncture

One of the major Oriental healing arts is acupuncture, which involves the insertion of needles at specific points on the body. These special points are located along the various meridians, twelve of which correspond to a particular organ. It is indeed an art as well as a science to be able to locate the precise point at which a needle should be inserted. If it is not placed in the right position, the procedure will not have the desired effect. The purpose of acupuncture is to move or restore the flow of *chi* through the insertion of the needles along the meridians relevant to the illness.

The needles are inserted quickly and left in place for several minutes. Sometimes the doctor will just pierce the skin, while other times the needle will be inserted up to an inch deep. The doctor might twirl the needle to increase stimulation. Another process of stimulating the acupuncture points is called *moxabustion*. In one method of moxabustion, the needles' heads are wrapped with dry *moxa* (Chinese wormwood) and burned. The needle conducts the heat into the acupuncture point. In yet another process, called electroacupuncture, the doctor connects each needle to a small machine that stimulates the needles with a low electrical pulse.

To those people raised with Western medical treatments, acupuncture is often viewed as a superstitious practice. The thought of having needles inserted into various regions of the body, even places as delicate as the face, can make even the staunchest Westerner squeamish. Those who have experienced acupuncture, however, claim that it is a painless, effective treatment for many illnesses. An acupuncture patient probably will feel a slight sensation when the needles are inserted. As the acupuncture works, the patient also might feel the presence of *chi* at the sites of the needles or the movement of *chi* in the body.

All this discussion about *chi* and influencing its movement through the body may be difficult for you to accept. Western scientists and doctors have devised several theories to explain why acupuncture works, especially when it is used to alleviate pain. One theory is based on the fact that the body produces endorphins and enkephalins, natural painkilling chemicals that also can help allergies and depression and can facilitate healing. Stimulating acupuncture points increases the body's production of endorphins and enkephalins. Another theory to explain acupuncture is that it has a placebo effect if the patient truly believes that it will help. Still another is based on the fact that some scientists and doctors feel that our vital energy is not *chi*, as the Chinese know it, but rather electricity. Acupuncture affects the way electricity travels along the meridians. Kirlian photography, which illustrates bioelectricity, provides evidence that this is a viable theory. The picture of a hand before and after acupuncture reveals an increased flow of electricity after the treatment. Finally, the gate theory of pain also is used to explain acupuncture. According to this theory, the body contains neuropathway "gates" along the spinal cord leading to the brain. Acupuncture closes the gates so that messages of pain do not reach the brain.

From a Chinese medicine point of view, acupuncture works as a result of regulating the flow of *chi* and blood. There is a Chinese expression, "There is no pain if there is free flow; if there is pain, there is no free flow."

Acupuncture has been shown to be an effective analgesic and has even been used instead of anesthetics during surgery. The stimulation of the acupuncture points in order to produce an analgesic effect causes the brain to release endorphins, which are the body's natural painkilling chemicals. Although Chinese doctors might use anesthetics during an operation, using acupuncture as an analgesic necessitates using only a fraction of the dose that a surgical patient in the West would receive. This is especially important for people who are sensitive to painkillers and anesthesia, as acupuncture is a harmless, safe way to treat pain.

Acupuncture can be an effective treatment for both terminal and nonterminal illnesses. A therapy that can be used alone or in combination with another treatment, it is also useful in dealing with the side effects of conventional medicine.

If you are considering acupuncture as a healing therapy, try to get a referral from an acupuncture society or school, from the pain clinic at your local hospital, or from someone who has experienced the treatment firsthand. Investigate the training and experience of the doctor until you are satisfied with his or her qualifications. Licensing varies by state: Some license independent practitioners, while others restrict practice to medical doctors (those with an M.D. degree) or allow acupuncturists to work only under such a doctor's supervision. Contact the American Association of Acupuncture and Oriental Medicine, the National Commission for the Certification of Acupuncturists, or the National Accreditation Commission for Schools and Colleges of Acupuncture and Oriental Medicine (see the Natural Medicine Resources section) for information regarding licensing requirements in your state and for more information about acupuncture.

Visits to an acupuncturist range in cost from $35 to $75. Some insurance companies do cover the cost of acupuncture, but many still do not, and some will cover only those treatments recommended by a conventional doctor. Be sure to check your policy regarding your coverage for acupuncture.

When you visit an acupuncturist, make sure that the doctor uses either presterilized disposable needles or an autoclave, which is a sterilizing machine. An autoclave is the only effective way to sterilize needles and other medical or dental instruments sufficiently.

To many people in the West, acupuncture is a strange procedure, of which they are skeptical. It is an art and a science that has been practiced for thousands of years, however, and its effects and benefits are often not acknowledged by orthodox Western medicine.

Acupressure

Acupressure is a therapy that is similar to acupuncture in that it uses the same geography of meridians and acupuncture (or acupressure) points. Instead of using needles, however, hands or feet gently pressure the appropriate points. Acupressure relaxes tense muscles, improves blood circulation, and stimulates the body's ability to heal itself.

Acupressure, which predates acupuncture, was developed approximately five thousand years ago by the Chinese. They discovered that pressing certain points on the body not only relieved localized pain, but could affect other parts of the body and internal organs as well. Acupressure was increasingly disregarded, however, as the Chinese began to use needles to stimulate the acupressure points.

Acupressure points are illustrated in the figures on pages 373–76. The descriptions of treatments for various conditions will refer to these diagrams and name the corresponding numbers that are relevant to use. For example, in treating migraine headaches, the text will read: "GB 20, located below the base of the skull in the hollows between the vertical neck muscles." Once you locate the point on yourself or the person you are treating, apply firm and steady pressure. It will take practice and experimentation to find the points and pressure that work for you.

Acupressure is not intended to cure serious illness or replace orthodox medical treatments for those illnesses. It can, however, increase relaxation, improve circulation, and ease pain, thereby maximizing health. Since it utilizes the same points as in acupuncture, specific *chi* or blood regulating or nourishing benefits associated with the points can be realized. It is an inexpensive and simple therapy to learn and one that, if practiced correctly, is entirely safe.

Here are some tips to bear in mind when administering acupressure to yourself or others:

- Use only gentle pressure; it should not cause any pain.
- Since there are a number of acupoints that are forbidden during pregnancy, you should work on a pregnant woman only under the instruction of a qualified acupuncture or acupressure practitioner.
- Do not use acupressure on someone who is taking drugs or alcohol.
- Do not administer acupressure immediately after eating.
- It is best for the patient to sit or lie down, as he or she may feel drowsy during a procedure.

Movement and Meditation

Advocates of Oriental medicine also believe that you can heal yourself through the dedicated practice of different kinds of movement and meditation.

The martial arts are different forms of exercise that require and develop supreme control, discipline, and strength in the individual. A gentle martial art, tai chi chuan, can help a person develop inner strength and control. The Chinese believe that movement is essential for the human body. Tai chi chuan involves slow, deliberate movements, a sense of communion with nature, and concentration on finding one's *chi*. The philosophy is that if one can locate one's *chi* and learn how to use it, one can maintain good health. Some martial arts schools offer classes in tai chi chuan, and it is an exercise that requires many years of dedicated practice to develop fully.

Another form of meditation, called chi-gong, is also used to find one's *chi*. Chinese doctors believe that a ball of *chi* is located in the abdominal or pelvic region, and through meditation people can learn to move their *chi* to the appropriate areas of their body. The idea, again, is to learn to influence the flow of *chi* so as to maintain its balance in the body.

Even when you are working with a doctor or trying to heal yourself, all Oriental medicine seems to require willing and dedicated participation on your part. Oriental medicine has been practiced for thousands of years, and it is effective. Of course, as with any healing treatment, not all forms will work in every case or all of the time. Oriental medicine does seem to substantiate, however, the connection of the mental and physical. This belief is inherent in the Eastern philosophy of health, and it is utilized to treat illness and to maximize health.

HOMEOPATHY

Homeopathy is a system of health care and treatment that was developed in the 1800s by Dr. Samuel Hahnemann. The philosophy of homeopathy is holistic, viewing the individual as a totality of interdependent parts and working from the notion that the mental and physical realms are inseparable. Hahnemann believed that orthodox medicine was a system of "contraries," meaning that doctors treated the symptoms of an illness by using drugs that oppose, or suppress, them. He began to call conventional medicine *allopathic,* meaning "different" and "disease, suffering." Hahnemann recognized that removing or masking symptoms did not treat the underlying cause of the illness, which could, in effect, develop into a more serious condition.

In homeopathy, symptoms are seen as a healthy response of the body's defense mechanism. The vital force, or vital energy, acts to keep the body in balance. When the body is threatened by some harmful external influence, the vital force (or defense mechanism) produces symptoms in its struggle against the harmful agent. Therefore, to a homeopathic doctor, fever is a sign that the body is fighting illness. A cough, which an allopathic doctor would try to suppress with medication, is seen by the homeopath as the natural way to expel mucus from the body. Bear in mind that this does not mean you must suffer with coughing all day long. You can use herbal cough drops and drink teas with honey, for example, to soothe your throat. However, if you are not willing to endure some discomfort during your sickness, you should reassess whether natural medicine treatments are appropriate for you.

Believing that drug prescriptions for specific illnesses often were based on an inadequate understanding of the drugs and their effects, Hahnemann began to test, or "prove," drugs on healthy women and men, including himself, to determine their effects. He tested remedies on people rather than animals because he knew that people usually react differently than animals do. This human testing is possible because the homeopathic remedies are nontoxic. In more than two hundred years of using the homeopathic formulations, there has been no reported case of a permanent adverse reaction.

In his provings, Hahnemann discovered that each remedy induced particular symptoms in a healthy person. When that remedy was given to a sick person exhibiting those same symptoms, it helped cure the person. Based on this notion that like cures like, Hahnemann formulated the Law of Similars. It states that a substance causing certain symptoms in a healthy person can cure a sick person with the same symptoms. The theory behind the Law of Similars is that the body enlists its own energies to heal itself and defend against illness. If a substance that causes a similar response in terms of similar symptoms is administered, the body steps up its fight against it, thereby promoting cure.

In an attempt to lessen the initial aggravating effects that remedies sometimes had on patients, Hahnemann administered very small dosages. Ironically, he discovered that the smaller the dose, the more powerful the effect. This led him to develop the Law of Infinitesimals, which states that the smaller the dose, the more effective it is in stimulating the body to respond against the illness.

In order to prepare smaller and smaller doses, Hahnemann would put a substance through a series of dilutions. He would begin with the original substance, putting one part in nine parts of an 87 percent solution of alcohol and distilled water. He then subjected to *succussion,* or vigorously agitated, the vial by striking it one hundred times against a leather pad. Hahnemann believed that subjecting the substance to succussion activated the therapeutic potential of it. This first step yields a one-in-ten dilution, also indicated as a "1× dilution." Hahnemann would then take one part of this 1× dilution and put it in nine parts of diluent, subjecting it to succussion to yield a 2× dilution. This process, referred to as the Law of Potentization, could continue indefinitely, producing increasingly potent dosages.

Hahnemann believed in administering one homeopathic remedy at a time in order to establish its effects. He treated all patients as whole people, taking their symptoms as part of their whole being rather than treating them separately, and apart from the rest of the person. This method differs from orthodox medicine in which specialists treat specific illnesses and body parts, and patients often take many drugs simultaneously.

Homeopathy views health as a state of freedom and well-being on three interdependent levels: physical, emotional, and mental. The most serious symptoms usually affect the deeper parts of a person; therefore, it is most important to treat the mental state, then the emotional, and finally the physical. This is in keeping with the holistic view of natural medicine, which treats the entire person—physically and mentally. In other words, a homeopath would say that it is not enough to treat you for migraine headaches, because if the stressors producing the migraines are not addressed, the migraines will recur or other symptoms could develop.

The German homeopath, Constantine Hering, who emigrated to the United States in the 1830s, recorded the changes in posttreatment symptoms. Based on his findings that healing occurs from the inside out, he laid the groundwork for Hering's Law of Cure, which is recognized not only by homeopaths but by acupuncturists and psychotherapists as well.

Hering's Law states that cure occurs from within outward, from the most vital to the least important organs. The body deals with the most significant aspect of the condition first, shifting during treatment to the next most important aspect, and so on. For instance, healing is believed to be in progress—from the inside out—if your chest pains subside but a skin rash develops. During homeopathic treatment, your condition can change so that the same or other remedies may be needed to facilitate the entire process of cure.

Hering's Law further states that symptoms will appear and disappear in the reverse order in which they originally appeared. The patient may also reexperience symptoms from a past condition. According to Hering, healing often begins with the upper body parts and descends. Therefore, if chronic headaches subside but stiff fingers are felt, the homeopath might believe that healing is taking place, and gradually the fingers should return to normal. At times, healing may not follow the traditional pattern of Hering's Law, but as long as the patient feels stronger and is improved overall, it is safe to assume that the treatment is working.

Based on the order "first, do no harm," homeopathy is a safe and effective system of treating many common acute and chronic ailments. For a temporary, minor, self-limited illness or injury, you probably can treat yourself with homeopathic remedies after consulting with your doctor. You can obtain remedies from homeopathic pharmacists, or even from some drugstores or health-food stores. For a more chronic, persistent illness, you should consult a qualified homeopathic practitioner. Professional homeopathic medical doctors graduate from conventional four-year medical schools with a Doctor of Medicine (M.D.) degree and often complete postgraduate training in homeopathy to learn this holistic specialty. Homeopathic schools can be found worldwide, but to master the art and science of the system, physicians often learn from experienced homeopathic doctors. The fees charged by homeopaths vary, as does insurance coverage. Some states and insurance companies honor homeopathic treatment and some do not, and some will cover it only if it is performed by a licensed medical doctor.

HYDROTHERAPY

Sometimes the most obvious and simplest remedies are the ones most often overlooked. Consider water—it composes two-thirds of our bodies and covers four-fifths of the earth's surface. Human beings can survive for weeks without food but only a few days without water. How can an element so common and abundant possibly be useful in healing?

The use that probably comes to mind first is the practice of swimming as physical therapy or bathing in a whirlpool to soothe sore muscles. But water has other healthful benefits as well, and in its various forms it can even be used to treat injuries and illnesses. It can work on the whole body, as in a bath, or on one area, as in the use of a compress. Water benefits the entire body by reenergizing it. Using a water therapy on one body part also can affect another beneficially, such as the use of a hot footbath to aid decongestion. Every organ and cell requires water, which helps nourish, detoxify, and maintain the right temperature of the body.

One of the earliest records of the therapeutic use of water dates back to the Greek god of medicine known as Aesculapius. At his temples, bathing and massage were used as a form of cure. Hippocrates also used water therapeutically. He advocated drinking water to alleviate fever, and he believed that baths could fight sickness. The Greek doctor Galen, who wrote Rome's outstanding medical text, also believed baths, both hot and cold, had beneficial effects, as did the Greek medical writer Celsus. Of course, this is true, because, in fact, one of the major reasons that health has increased over the ages is that sanitation and hygiene have improved.

In the eighteenth century, German, English, and Italian clergy revived the therapeutic use of water. In 1797, a Scottish doctor, James Currie, wrote a book called *Medical Reports on the Effects of Water, Cold and Warm, as a Remedy in Fever and Febrile Diseases*. In the early nineteenth century, Vincent Preissnitz, a Silesian farmer, reinvented water therapy using methods such as dousings, showers, immersions, and single and double compresses. His procedures spread to England, Germany, and Scandinavia, as well as the United States.

Later in the nineteenth century, Sebastian Kniepp

adapted Preissnitz's techniques into his own theories of hydrotherapy. Kniepp, born in Bavaria in 1821, was a frail and sickly person. After reading a pamphlet about water cures, he decided to plunge into an icy cold river in the middle of winter with the hope that it would cure his ailments. Kniepp jumped into the river every day, and although it might seem absurd, he claimed that over time he became physically stronger. Along with Preissnitz's techniques, Kniepp claimed that walking in cold water or on wet grass was therapeutic.

Hydrotherapy is based on the law of action and reaction. If the skin is heated, either by a hot bath or compress, blood is immediately drawn to the surface and then returns to the deeper blood vessels. Likewise, cold water will drive blood away from the surface, but will cause a secondary effect of warmth as the blood returns to the tissues and vessels from which it was pushed away. This concept of immediate action followed by a secondary and more lasting reaction is a basic principle of hydrotherapy.

The different forms and temperatures of water have different physical and chemical effects on the body. Cold water is essentially restorative and reenergizing. It can reduce fever, act as a diuretic and anesthetic, alleviate pain, help relieve constipation, and eliminate toxins from the body. Ice and ice water can relieve the pain of burns, help control bleeding, and reduce swelling from injury. Warm water, in contrast, has a relaxing effect. Hot baths induce perspiration, which is essential in eliminating toxins from the body. Hot compresses and baths can reduce pain and inflammation, although cold water should be used for inflammation due to injury. This is important because hot water increases blood flow and would thereby increase inflammation in an injury. Alternating hot and cold baths can help increase circulation. Steam is a form of hydrotherapy that opens pores, increases perspiration, and sometimes alleviates chest congestion. Humidifying air is good for those who suffer from sinus conditions and airborne allergies.

Water has therapeutic uses when used internally or externally, at varying degrees of temperatures and pressures, and in its three forms: ice, liquid, or steam. Ice can be used as an anesthetic to chill the skin and dull pain. Boiling water is an antiseptic that can cleanse food and clothing. Hot compresses placed on the abdomen and herbal teas can work as antispasmodics to relieve cramps. If you need a diuretic, try drinking ice water or herbal tea or applying a hot, moist compress on your lower back; these all affect the kidneys to increase urine production. Colon irrigation, enemas, genital irrigation, the drinking of water, the taking of a sauna or hot baths all help to eliminate toxins. Drinking an emetic, such as salt water, can induce vomiting in order to expel certain poisonous substances. Finally, hot or cold baths or showers, whirlpools, and salt baths have a stimulating effect, while warm showers or herbal baths can act as a sedative.

Many different types of water application are used in hydrotherapy. Local heat can be achieved with a moist, hot compress or hot-water bottle; local cold requires a cold compress, frozen bandage, or ice pack or bag. A cold double compress is a cold compress covered with a dry cloth, such as wool or flannel, which creates internal heat. A pack is a larger form of the double compress, or it can be a clay, mustard, or flaxseed poultice. Alcohol, water, or witch hazel can be used in sponging, and you can achieve tonic friction by rubbing with a sponge or washcloth. Therapeutic showers can alternate between hot and cold, and the pressure of the shower can vary. Steam is therapeutic too, from a sauna, vaporizer, or humidifier.

One of the most common and most appreciated hydrotherapy techniques is the bath, a total immersion of either the body or a part of the body, such as hands, feet, arms, eyes, or fingers. Depending on the ailment you wish to treat, baths can be cold, tepid, or hot, can be long or short in duration, and can involve massage using a sponge, bath mitten, or loofah brush to create tonic friction. Baths can consist of plain water or contain salts, herbs, oatmeal, or mud. Following is a list of bath additives and their therapeutic benefits:

Apple cider vinegar: Fights fatigue; relieves sunburn and itchy skin.

Borax/cornstarch/bicarbonate of soda: Good antiseptic.

Bran: Softens skin and relieves itchiness.

Chamomile: Soothes skin and opens pores; helps to relieve insomnia and digestive problems.

Dead Sea salts: Restores body after injury.

Epsom salts: Increases perspiration, relaxes muscles, and helps to relieve catarrh.

Fennel/nettle: Helps to rid skin of impurities.

Ginger powder: Relaxes muscles, tones skin, and increases circulation. (Use in small amounts as it is very powerful.)

Hayflower/oatstraw: Helps to rid skin of impurities.

Nutmeg: Increases perspiration.

Oatmeal: Good for skin problems, such as itchiness, hives, windburn, and sunburn.

Pine: Increases perspiration, softens skin, and relieves rashes.

Rosemary: Stimulates blood circulation.

Sage: Stimulates sweat glands.

Salt: Promotes a relaxing effect.

Sulphur: Good antiseptic and helps to rid skin of parasites; helps relieve acne.

It is easy and inexpensive to treat yourself to a wide variety of baths. Most of the listed herbs and preparations can be bought in drugstores, herbal pharmacies, health-food stores, or through catalogs. Remember to purchase them in small quantities since they lose their potency in approximately one year.

BOTANICAL MEDICINE

Botanical medicine, also referred to as herbalism, plant healing, physiomedicalism, medical herbalism, and phytotherapy, uses remedies made from plants called herbs. Whereas botanists define herbs as any plants that do not contain woody fibers, medicinal herbalists define them as any plant that has healing properties. Herbal remedies can also come from trees, ferns, seaweeds, or lichens, and herbalists will use whole plants, rather than isolating the principal active compounds from them. Whole plants contain proteins, enzymes, vitamins, minerals, and other trace elements that readily assimilate in the body. In fact, the three fatty acids essential for life—linoleic, linolenic, and arachidonic—are all found in plants. Botanical medicine is a safe and natural way to treat specific ailments and assist recuperation from illness in order to restore physiological balance.

The history of botanical medicine goes back through the ages, with "recipes" for herbal remedies being passed from generation to generation. Plants are natural agents of cure, and animals have an instinct for their curative powers. You've probably seen a dog nibble on grass. No, he doesn't think he's part goat—but he might have a belly-ache and is eating the grass to aid his digestion. For centuries, Native Americans have chewed willow-tree bark to cure headaches. The bark contains salicylic acid, the active ingredient in aspirin.

Traditional herbal medicine originated in ancient times in India, China, and Egypt, with the earliest records appearing in Egypt and Assyria. Many of the plants listed in these and in Greek documents are still used today. Over time, herbalists have compiled classifications—descriptions of plants arranged according to their medicinal properties. Today, there are more than 750,000 plants in the world, and only a small percentage have been evaluated. The World Health Organization investigates and supports herbal medicine throughout the world in order to learn more about this natural method of healing.

Plants are used not only in botanical medicine but in allopathic medicine as well, and once served as the basis for nearly all drugs. In order to appreciate the benefits of botanical medicine, it is useful to look at how allopathy has used plants in preparing drugs.

Until the 1800s, most drugs were given by mouth in the form of ground leaves, roots, or flowers, or in teas, tinctures, or extracts. Doctors studied botany as a matter of course, and herbalists without medical training, particularly women, also flourished.

Prior to the 1800s, there was no standard clinical evidence on which doctors could base their selection of drugs for treatment. In 1803, a German pharmacist isolated morphine from opium, signifying the first time that a pure active principle had been obtained from a crude plant drug. With this pure form of morphine, doctors could give exact doses, knowing their effects. In the mid-nineteenth century, there was a push to isolate pure forms of active principles from medicinal plants. By 1870, caffeine had been isolated from coffee, nicotine from tobacco, and cocaine from coca.

These isolated compounds are generally more toxic than the whole plants from which they are derived. Scientists and doctors believed it was better to treat patients with the purified drug, and they disregarded other compounds in the plant. Herbalists, however, recognized that the whole plant has a different effect from the isolated substance since it contains many other vital ingredients that interact to give an overall effect.

Besides using isolated principles, chemists also experiment with molecules to synthesize new drugs. Their goal usually is to increase the potency and efficacy of the drug. More potent drugs can be risky, however, given that doctors often prescribe numerous medications simultaneously. And some drugs are so potent as to be addictive. Adverse drug reactions, or side effects, are the most common effects of iatrogenic (doctor-caused) illness.

Many commonly used drugs are derived from plants. For instance, digitoxin comes from foxglove (*Digitalis purpurea*) and is prescribed for heart failure; atropine is from deadly nightshade (*Atropa belladonna*) and dilates pupils; morphine comes from the opium poppy (*Papaver somniferum*) and is a powerful painkiller.

Herbalists may use the root, rhizome, stem, leaf, flower, seed, fruit, bark, wood, resin, or whole plant in preparing an herbal medication. Familiar with the interaction of various plants with each other, herbalists usually will use several plants or extracts in one preparation, since they can sometimes be more effective when combined than when used separately. Plants contain oils, alkaloids (nitrogen compounds), tannins, resins, fats, carbohydrates, proteins, and enzymes that all contribute to their medicinal action. Each substance has a function and can support, control, or otherwise affect the other constituents. In using the whole plant, the herbalist will get the most gentle, safe, and effective benefit from the treatment.

Herbal remedies can be taken in the form of tablets, capsules, lotions, ointments, suppositories, inhalants, or teas and juices. For herbal drinks, the basic proportion is 1 ounce (25 grams) herbs to 1 pint (0.5 liter) liquid. Herb teas will keep for three days in a tightly covered container in the refrigerator. Following is a list of common terms referring to botanical medications:

Carminative: Relieves flatulence, colic.

Cholagogue: Stimulates release of bile from the gallbladder.

Decoction: Drink made from roots, bark, or berries simmered in boiling water and strained.

Demulcent: Soothing substance for the skin.

Emmenagogue: Stimulates menstruation.

Emollient: Used internally to soothe membranes or externally to soften skin.

Infusion: Boiling water is poured over leaves, flowers, or the whole plant (excluding seeds and berries).

Nervine: That which is calming.

Ointments: Applied externally; effective for skin conditions.

Poultice: Crushed plant and hot water mixed to produce a paste that is wrapped in a thin cloth and applied to the skin.

Pressed juice: Juice from fresh plants is rich in vitamins and minerals; can be used in tinctures or diluted in water.

Teas: Made from pouring boiling water over

fermented leaves or stalks from one or more plants; fermentation produces tannin; premade teabags can be purchased.

Tinctures: One part herb in five parts of diluted alcohol.

Tisane: Add boiling water to fresh or dried plant, usually green leaves.

You can dry your own leaves by laying them on a wire rack in a warm, dry place for forty-eight hours; store in airtight glass containers. This should keep for one year. When preparing a tisane, use a separate pot from tea, as tannin will interfere with the tisane remedy.

Vulnerary: Used to treat and heal wounds.

An herbalist can give you information as to appropriate herbs used to treat various symptoms. A consultation with an herbalist is similar to one with other natural healers. The herbalist will check your heart and pulse, physical symptoms, and perhaps perform some laboratory tests, such as blood and urine analyses. More important, the herbal practitioner will spend quite some time observing, talking, questioning, and listening to you in order to determine the imbalance and disharmony of your body and life.

If you find a satisfactory course of treatment with a particular herbalist, it is good to stay with that person so as not to disrupt the healing process. Sometimes symptoms are aggravated before healing occurs, and some people and certain disorders take longer to heal than others. Patience and willing participation in your treatment is essential in order to maximize the benefits of botanical medicine. And any herbal treatment should be undertaken only in consultation with your physician.

PHYSICAL MEDICINE

Chiropractic

The word *chiropractic* means "treatment by the hands, or manipulation." It is a system of healing that was developed by David Daniel Palmer (1845–1913) in Iowa in 1895. Palmer believed that displacements of the spine caused pressure on nerves, which created pain or symptoms in other parts of the body.

Although chiropractic medicine subscribes to traditional concepts of anatomy and physiology, it differs from traditional medicine in that it is holistic, meaning it considers the patient as a whole, with an emphasis on body structure. Practitioners rely on X rays and standard orthopedic and neurological tests to diagnose problems, focusing on abnormalities of the spine. Treatment often involves direct thrust on specific vertebrae that are out of alignment, which helps to restore the flow of energy. Two terms that you will encounter in chiropractic are *adjustment* and *manipulation*. Adjustments involve dynamic thrusts (rapid, precise, and painless force) to a specific vertebra in order to remove any interference with nerves. It is not only the adjustment itself that is important, but the body's healing reaction to it. Manipulations are more general reorderings of bones to realign joints and increase the patient's range of motion.

Chiropractic is helpful in treating many conditions, including back pain and musculoskeletal disorders as well as certain systemic illnesses, such as asthma, migraines, and digestive problems. These systemic disorders, however, can be helped only if there is evidence of a structural and neurological involvement. Chiropractic treatment must be administered by a qualified and licensed professional, and it usually involves multiple visits in order to maintain proper spinal alignment. Initial visits can run from $50 to $150, with routine visits priced at approximately $50, and most insurance companies do provide coverage for this treatment. Chiropractors usually undergo at least two years of college plus an additional four years of professional education, and they must pass state and national licensing examinations.

Massage

The word *massage* derives from both the Greek *masso* ("knead") and the Arabic *mass* ("press gently"). It is a form of physical medicine that is completely harmless, comfortable, and relaxing. While a massage can be given by anyone, a trained massage therapist often seems to have a magic touch.

Massage works on the soft tissues, muscles, and ligaments of the body. It stimulates circulation and the function of the nervous system and helps to lower blood pressure. It can soothe muscle tension and headaches and can help relieve insomnia. Massage is particularly beneficial after exercise. During a workout, waste products build up in the muscles. It can take the lymphatic system days to wash them away. Massage speeds up this process by improving the circulation of blood and lymph.

There are two main types of massage: shiatsu and Swedish. Shiatsu was developed in Japan at about the same time that acupuncture began to flourish in China. This massage involves finger pressure that stimulates the acupuncture points along the body's meridians. One form of shiatsu firmly massages certain areas of the body to stimulate the flow of energy and restore balance. Another form involves the use of a single fingertip to stimulate acupuncture points. The purpose of shiatsu is to alter the flow of energy within the body, and it works along the same principle as acupuncture. Shiatsu therapists also emphasize the importance of good nutrition and positive mental outlook, and they encourage clients to make lifestyle changes that promote greater health. Shiatsu can be combined with chiropractic to maximize its healing effects.

Swedish massage, which is more common in the West, involves four essential techniques, with the underlying premise that the hands should not lose contact with the body. Swedish massage is effective because of its continual, rhythmic motions. These are the basic techniques.

Effleurage: Rhythmic stroking with open hands, with movements directed toward the heart; this motion soothes and relaxes the body.

Percussion: Brisk rhythmic movements with alternate hands that include cupping, hacking (with sides of hands), pummeling (with fists), clapping, and plucking; this stimulates the skin and circulation.

Petrissage: Deep movement that involves lifting, rolling, squeezing, and pressing the skin; this stimulates muscles and fatty tissues, stretching taut muscles to relax them.

Pressure: As the thumbs, fingertips, or heel of the hand make small pressured circular movements, friction stimulates superficial tissue.

When you visit a massage therapist, he or she probably will not take a detailed physical history, but you should inform him or her of any pains, illnesses, injuries, or recent surgeries you have had. The therapist usually will begin with the feet or back and will allow you a few moments to get used to the sensation of being touched and kneaded. It should be a thoroughly pleasurable treat!

Sessions are usually one hour long and cost approximately $30 to $70. Therapeutic massage is covered by some insurance companies when it is required by a doctor for the treatment of a particular ailment or injury due to an automobile or work-related accident. Massage is generally entirely safe, but you should not use it if the following conditions exist:

- Infectious, open wounds or bruises.
- Varicose veins.
- Fever.
- Inflamed joints or acute arthritis.
- Thrombosis or phlebitis (could disturb blood clot).

Reflexology

Reflexology is a technique of deeply massaging the soles of the feet in order to affect various parts of the body that are ailing. It was developed in China and India at the same time that acupuncture originated. Reflexology was brought to England in the twentieth century by Dr. William Fitzgerald, who called it zone therapy. In the United States Eunice Ingham developed Fitzgerald's teachings in the 1930s. Today, reflexology is growing in popularity, with schools located in Europe and the United States. Many practitioners of reflexology also perform chiropractic, osteopathy, and homeopathy.

Reflexology works on the premise that internal organs share the same nerve supplies as certain corresponding areas of the skin. Practitioners believe that the entire body is represented on the feet, primarily on the soles. By pressing the proper points on the feet, one can stimulate the organ associated with that point. These points are not the same as acupuncture points or meridians, many of which are not even represented on the feet.

During a reflexology session, the client will lie on a massage table while the practitioner feels the feet for granule-like substances deep within them. These "crystals" are actually waste deposits that build up in the nerve endings and capillaries and restrict the free flow of blood. The reflexology treatment breaks up the deposits so that they can be flushed from the body.

As the reflexologist "reads" the feet, he or she can determine which organs are affected. The patient will usually feel pain when a particular point is pressed, and sometimes in the corresponding organ or area of the body. The practitioner applies pressure with the edge of the thumb or finger and rotates it clockwise. The pressure is deep but should not be too painful. A session usually lasts from thirty to ninety minutes, and a client may require several sessions. Reflexology is beneficial for functional disorders that can be reversed, such as sinus problems, constipation, asthma, bladder problems, headaches, and stress.

PSYCHOTHERAPY

Psychotherapy, or "talk treatment," is an invaluable natural therapy for fostering and maintaining overall health. There has been much discussion in recent years about the mind-body connection. Although this has been an inherent part of holistic medicine throughout the world over time, orthodox Western medicine is realizing more and more the power of the mind and the importance of psychological treatments.

Mental health is important to physical health and vice versa. Emotional problems cause stress, which evokes physical symptoms and illness; physical illness, likewise, can cause a person to become depressed or lose energy and motivation. Doctors and patients are increasingly aware of the interplay of the mind and body and that in fact they may be inseparable, or one and the same.

Psychotherapy often requires you to talk about your feelings and problems, but it also can involve action, such as finding ways to alter your patterns of behavior. Treatment can be conducted on an individual basis between therapist and client, or it can be held within a group format. Group therapy allows clients to support and help each other, which can be just as valuable as receiving guidance from a therapist. People who seek out psychological treatment are not necessarily sick. They may simply be seeking greater understanding about themselves and their behavior.

There are many different kinds of psychotherapy, and some are more beneficial than others for treating particular disorders or problems. You may not hit upon the right therapy immediately, but don't give up. Success and progress in psychotherapy often take much time. If you really feel it's not working for you (and you've discussed this with the therapist), try a different therapist, and you might get better results. Psychotherapy, like many holistic, natural treatments, requires a willingness on the part of patients to be open to the treatment and to help themselves. You might go to a psychotherapist or counselor with the hope that the doctor will "cure" you. In fact, it takes work by both the therapist and the client in order for the treatment to be effective. The following sections list the major types of psychotherapy:

Supportive Psychotherapy

In this treatment, you can openly discuss your problems and feelings in a trusting, comfortable environment. The therapist should be a good listener who allows you the opportunity to vent your feelings and who may make suggestions or point out insights that will give you a sense of support, without the feeling of being judged.

Exploratory Psychotherapy

This kind of treatment encourages you to explore your problems and issues, rather than just airing them. The therapist is usually active in the discussion and will let you know if you are avoiding a particular issue. Many healthy people pursue exploratory therapy as a way of learning more about themselves or to deal with a particular issue or aspect of their lives that they feel needs resolving or improvement.

Psychoanalysis

This treatment, which was originated by Sigmund Freud at the turn of the century, has taken a variety of forms. In classical psychoanalysis, you lie on a couch and talk freely about feelings, dreams, or whatever comes to mind. The psychoanalyst interprets what you say in terms of your childhood experiences and relationship with your parents. Psychoanalysis is usually intensive and long-term.

Other forms of psychoanalytic treatment focus on how your early emotional experiences have affected your current feelings and perceptions of yourself and relationships. This kind of therapy can help free you from pent-up or repressed childhood anger, frustration, hurt, and dependency. By working through these feelings, you will gain a greater sense of self-understanding and self-esteem.

Gestalt Therapy

Introduced in the United States by Fritz Perls in the 1950s, this "humanistic" therapy believes that the present moment, not the past, is most important, and that every person is responsible for his or her actions and has the ability to change them. In a session, if something from the past is bothersome, the therapist will help you bring it into the present. Gestalt therapists use many techniques to increase your awareness of yourself in the moment. For instance, if you are crying in a session, the therapist might ask you to speak to your tears. Merely talking about them promotes greater distancing between yourself and your emotions. Another Gestalt technique is for you to behave in a session opposite from the way you feel. For example, if you are very shy, the therapist might ask you to act like an outgoing person. Doing this will allow you to become aware of a part of yourself that exists but has remained undeveloped or repressed.

Behavioral Therapy

Behavioral therapists believe that all behavior is learned either through conditioning or the reinforcement of specific actions. For instance, if your mother taught you when you were growing up that all animals are dirty, you might develop a fear of animals, such as dogs. When the behavior you learned is negative or maladaptive, adverse psychological symptoms (in this example, a phobia) can result. Behavioral therapy can teach you new ways of behaving to help you live a more positive, happy, and productive life.

Behavioral therapy can resolve phobias, sexual dysfunction, inhibitions, and increase self-assertiveness. The therapist will help you learn new behaviors to replace those that are maladaptive. One method is called *operant conditioning*, by which new behaviors are rewarded and undesirable ones are ignored. In the *modeling* technique, the therapist "models," or displays for you to copy, the new behavior you are to practice. *Systemic desensitization* is a step-by-step process to help relieve specific fears or inhibitions.

Cognitive Therapy

This therapy was developed by American psychologist Aaron Beck in the 1960s. *Cognition* refers to a person's thinking, perception, and memory. If the therapist views your cognition as the cause of your emotional problems, the therapy will try to alter your perceptions and thoughts about yourself in order to alleviate the symptoms or problems. For example, if you were constantly denigrated by your father when you were growing up, chances are you developed a low self-esteem and often feel worthless. A cognitive therapist would point out evidence to the contrary, emphasizing your achievements that prove your self-worth.

Couples Therapy

Those who are married or involved in a serious intimate relationship know that even the best relationships require work. In couples therapy, you can visit a therapist either together or separately in order to understand and resolve tensions that exist within your relationship. Therapy can be useful to both heterosexual and homosexual couples.

Family Therapy

Families are intricate, dynamic networks that often require an objective outsider to help clear the air or resolve conflicts. When one or more family members has a problem, it often throws the entire unit into crisis, and this is when therapy can be beneficial. A family therapist is able to observe how the family operates together and can help the members understand not only how to deal with each other, but their own roles within the family.

Just as it is important to find the right kind of therapy, it is equally important to build a good relationship with your therapist. As with other kinds of relationships, this can happen spontaneously, or it may take time. Within the emotional context of therapy, it is often difficult to discern how you feel about your therapist. Bear in mind that it is valid and important to discuss the feelings you have toward your therapist with him or her. This might reveal insight as to how you relate to others.

The different kinds of therapists are distinguished by their training. *Psychotherapist* is a general term that refers to anyone who practices psychotherapy. A *psychiatrist* is a medical doctor who is trained in psychotherapy and can prescribe drugs for treating mental disorders. A *clinical psychologist* holds a doctoral degree in psychology and has training in psychotherapy. He or she cannot prescribe medicine, and may specialize in a particular type of therapy, such as psychoanalytic, behavioral, and so on. A *psychoanalyst* is a psychiatrist or psychologist who is specially trained in psychoanalysis.

You can seek psychotherapy from a private therapist or from a mental health center or clinic. Fees vary according to the practitioner, though some are willing to use a sliding scale—that is, they will charge a fee based on your income and the amount you are able to afford. Some insurance policies provide a psychotherapy benefit, while others do not. If your policy does, find out whether there is a limit to the number of sessions or if there is a cap on the amount of coverage provided each year.

BIOFEEDBACK

Biofeedback probably presents the greatest evidence of the mind's influence over the body. In a healthy person, physiological functions are performed and regulated by the brain and central nervous system. The mind, however, often interferes, such as under conditions of stress that produce tension in the body. Biofeedback can teach the patient to intervene under these conditions in order to restore balanced functioning in the body.

Conscious control can affect many body functions that can be measured accurately and continuously, such as heart rate, skin temperature, blood pressure, muscle tension, and brain waves. The biofeedback equipment that measures these functions includes the electroencephalograph (EEG), which records nerve and brain waves, the electromyograph (EMG), which registers muscle tension, and the galvanic skin resistance instrument (GSR), which detects the electrical conductivity of the skin to record states of arousal, excitement, or nervousness.

When you are hooked up to these machines, they convey information to you through signals that can be recognized and interpreted easily. For instance, when the instrument detects muscle tension, a red light might go on or a certain sound might be emitted to signal what is happening to you internally. You then can use this information, in addition to certain relaxation and imagery techniques, to begin controlling the muscle tension. The techniques that are used in combination with the biofeedback equipment include relaxation and autosuggestion exercises, visual imagery, and meditation. For example, if the equipment signals that your heart rate is increasing, you can use imagery, by imagining a calm, peaceful place, or meditate through the repeating of a mantra in order to relax your mind and body. In biofeedback treatment, therefore, the patient is not the object of the therapy, he or she *becomes* the therapy itself.

There are many applications for biofeedback, including stress-related illness, neuromuscular problems, and personal growth and increased self-awareness. Biofeedback can be effective treatment for emotional or behavioral problems, such as anxiety, depression, phobias, insomnia, tension headaches, and bruxism (teeth-grinding). It also can be used to treat illnesses considered by some professionals to be psychosomatic such as asthma, ulcers, colitis, diarrhea, cardiac arrhythmia, hypertension, Raynaud's syndrome, and migraines. Biofeedback can help victims of stroke, cerebral palsy, and muscle spasms in some functions of the muscles and movement. Since biofeedback increases your recognition and understanding of your total mind-body functioning, it also can be beneficial in enhancing personal growth and self-awareness.

Many general and psychiatric hospitals have biofeedback clinics, and it is probably best to undergo treatments administered by a psychologist who is trained in biofeedback. A psychologist would be helpful in the process of developing greater self-awareness, and you might even consider combining biofeedback with psychotherapy.

When you begin biofeedback sessions, you should be informed about the equipment being used and the learning process and receive information about the muscles and the physiological functions involved in the treatment. Having this knowledge will help you to relax during the treatment and will probably enhance its success. Remember that while you must be an active participant in biofeedback, too much effort can produce unwanted stress. The key is to relax, using meditation, imagery, and other techniques, in order to focus fully on your internal states.

Biofeedback training can last weeks, months, or years, depending on your problem. Most people need at least six weeks' worth of sessions, which last from thirty to sixty minutes and can occur once a week or daily, again, depending on the need. The cost of biofeedback varies depending on your location, with an average cost of $75 per session. Check your insurance plan for coverage. You must learn to transfer what you learn from the biofeedback sessions to your daily life. It will take practice to begin to recognize the signs of trouble—such as muscle tension, headaches, and so on—and the situations in which they occur, and then to use the techniques that can relieve them without the biofeedback instrument. You probably will need periodic checkups in order to maintain the progress you have made.

NUTRITION

The value of good nutrition may be obvious, but it is often the obvious that is overlooked. If you do not eat the right foods, the organs and cells of your body will not get the nutrients they need to function and grow properly. Since food is a basic necessity, it also has been looked upon as essential medicine from very early times. People in ancient Greece and Egypt, for example, used garlic as a cure for respiratory infections, intestinal viruses, and skin conditions. Cabbage was a remedy for ulcers and headaches. In the 1700s, English ships began to carry lemons and limes to treat scurvy, a condition that affected sailors. It wasn't until the 1900s that scientists discovered the actual substance in citrus fruit that prevented scurvy. By this time, vitamin C had been isolated from lemons, and the first fat-soluble vitamin, A, was discovered.

By the 1940s, forty nutrients and thirteen vitamins had been isolated from foods. With the 1950s and 1960s came the era of processed foods, including the booming fast-food industry. This was followed in the next two decades by numerous fad diets as people desperately tried various ways to get rid of the weight gain that comes with this convenience.

Today, it seems that the public has a greater awareness of the kinds of things they ingest. New information on the dangers of substances such as pesticides, food additives, and saturated fats—and the benefits of nutrients—have altered the way many people eat. As you revamp your diet, however, it is important to read as much as you can in order to make informed choices about what you eat. Sometimes it is difficult to discern what is the latest fad and what is sound advice. Dieticians and nutritionists can help tailor your diet to your needs if you wish to pursue nutritional therapy to treat illness or allergies, or to bolster your health.

Essential Nutrients

All food is composed of certain substances that are necessary to maintain health: fats, proteins, carbohydrates, vitamins, minerals, and trace elements. Foods are characterized by categories (fat, carbohydrate, protein, dietary fiber), and a healthy diet balances a combination of them.

Protein Approximately 17 percent of your body is composed of protein, including muscle, hair, bone, nails, and skin. Protein is also necessary for the production of hormones and enzymes. Since protein cannot be stored in the body, it must be absorbed regularly from foods such as milk, yogurt, cheese, eggs, meat, fish, sprouts, nuts, seeds, and legumes. If you do not eat enough protein, your muscles and tissues will degenerate. Too much protein, however, could strain the liver and kidneys and disrupts the balance of minerals in your body. Protein should account for approximately 5 percent of your total caloric intake each day.

Fats Fat is an important source of energy. It helps to maintain organs, cell structure, nerves, and body temperature. Fat also carries fat-soluble vitamins, such as A, D, E, and K, around the body. There are three types of fatty acid: *saturated fat* primarily comes from animal sources, such as meat, fish, butter, cheese, eggs, and cream; *polyunsaturated fat* comes from plant sources, such as wheat germ and safflower, corn, and sunflower oils; *monounsaturated fat* is found in olive oil, avocados, and peanuts. Saturated fats, which can increase cholesterol levels, are the worst kinds of fat to consume. Most people in our society would probably benefit from reducing their overall fat intake. Fat should constitute no more than 30 percent of your total daily caloric intake, with only 10 percent of this coming from saturated fats.

Carbohydrates Our main source of energy is carbohydrates, which are converted into the glucose and glycogen that fuel muscles, the brain, and the nervous system. Carbohydrates come from starches and sugars. The best are starches in grains, legumes, and pastas, and sugars in fruits and vegetables. Refined sugar and flour contain high-calorie carbohydrates with little nutritional value. Unlike natural starches and sugars, which convert into glucose more slowly and are absorbed at a steady pace over time, they are absorbed quickly for instant bursts of energy. Carbohydrates should constitute the balance of your daily caloric intake (about 60 percent).

Dietary Fiber Fiber, also referred to as roughage, is an indigestible substance found naturally in cereals, beans, nuts, vegetables, and fruits. Containing no nutrients and remaining undigested, it moves through the intestinal tract. As it absorbs liquid, it helps produce large soft stools that are easily passed. Fiber helps speed the passage of waste through the bowel and helps to remove toxic substances from the body. Low-fiber foods can take three or four days to pass through the digestive tract; high-fiber foods, in contrast, are usually passed within twenty-four hours. By consuming an adequate amount of fiber—and thus helping to move waste through the bowel more quickly—you may reduce your chances of developing colon cancer, diverticular disease, and gallstones.

Fiber occurs naturally in a wide variety of foods. Whole-grain cereals; whole-wheat, or bulgar-wheat, products; brown rice; barley; and bran are excellent sources of roughage. Legumes, oats, barley, and rye are also good sources and they form substances that restrict the amount of fat and sugar the body absorbs. This can help lower blood cholesterol levels and blood pressure. Corn, apples, carrots, brussels sprouts, eggplant, celery, potatoes, peas, and dried fruit are all good sources of dietary fiber. You should consume approximately one and one-half to two ounces (forty to sixty grams) of fiber each day.

Vitamins/Minerals   Vitamins and minerals are essential in aiding metabolism and the chemical processes in the body that release energy from food. The thirteen major vitamins are A, C, D, E, K, and eight B vitamins, often referred to as the B complex. Vitamins are soluble in either water or fat. Vitamin C and most of the B vitamins are water soluble. They must be consumed each day since they cannot be stored in the body. Any excess C or B vitamins are excreted. Vitamins A, D, E, and K are fat soluble, and they can be stored in the body's fatty tissues. Vitamin B_{12} can be stored in the liver.

Vitamins and minerals often work together and interact

with each other. For example, vitamin C enhances the absorption of iron in the body. It is best to eat the daily required amounts of each vitamin and mineral in food.

If you decide to consult a nutritionist or dietician, he or she will help you devise a balanced diet and will recommend the supplements you should take according to any deficiencies you might have. If you are creating your own nutritional plan—or just modifying your eating habits— you should take a multivitamin and mineral supplement every day. This will ensure that you are getting the adequate amounts of nutrients that your body needs.

A Healthy Diet

Whole foods, or those produced with a minimal amount of processing, contain many of their original nutrients. Try to eat organically grown fruits and vegetables that have not been subject to chemical pesticides, meat and poultry that has not been given growth-hormone injections, and eggs from free-range chickens.

Generally, most people in our society need to eat more fruits and vegetables and to consume more fiber. It is best to eat fruits and vegetables raw and with their skins to ensure that you are getting all of their vitamins and minerals. Make sure to clean the skin thoroughly by scrubbing it with a brush (either a vegetable or pot-scrubbing brush) under running water to wash away unabsorbed chemicals from pesticides or other impurities. Fruits and vegetables should be eaten fresh, as they lose nutrients with age. They also lose nutrients through cooking, so try to cook them for as short a time and with as little liquid as possible. For example, if you usually boil vegetables, try steaming them instead. You'll probably enjoy their crispy texture and find that they have more taste! If you do boil your vegetables, consider using the liquid in stocks or sauces so as not to waste the vital nutrients.

Most of us also need to eat more fiber. If you now use white bread, try switching to whole-grain breads and cereals. Increase your fiber intake gradually in order to avoid a bloated feeling, which may occur temporarily.

If you want to consume less fat, eat only lean red meat in modest portions, and cook more poultry and fish. There are many good-quality low-fat products on the market, such as low-fat margarine. But use common sense in planning your diet. Remember that it is better to use just a little butter, a natural product, than to eat a lot of margarine, which contains added chemicals and hydrogenated fats. You also should consider using skim milk and low-fat yogurt and cheese. Avoid eating rich desserts, such as ice cream or pastries, fried foods, and rich sauces.

Most of us can probably do with less sugar and salt in our diets. Refined white sugar has no nutritional value, so try cutting down your use of it. If your sweet tooth will not be denied, replace sugar with honey or fruit juices—they are natural sweeteners. Try eating fruit or sugarless baked goods and jams that are sweetened only with fruit juices.

Although some salt is necessary, most people consume too much of it since it is used in excess in many processed foods. Remember, salt occurs naturally in many foods, so there is no reason to add more. Substitute herbs and spices for salt when you are cooking, and try to eat fewer processed foods. Generally, you should consume one ounce (twenty-five grams) or less of sugar and less than one-fourth ounce (six grams) of salt each day.

It was discovered long ago that honey and salt could help preserve foods. Over the past few decades, the use of artificial additives and preservatives has increased greatly, replacing the natural ones. Some of these are harmless in small amounts, and some additives even occur naturally, such as monosodium glutamate (MSG) in fermented soy products (soy sauce). However, when restaurants add excess amounts of MSG in the preparation of food, some people experience adverse physical symptoms, such as headaches, nausea, and dizziness.

Dyes, preservatives, stabilizers, antioxidants, and emulsifiers are all food additives that can cause reactions in people who are sensitive to these substances. Most additives are thoroughly tested for safety, and they must be listed on each product, according to the rules of the Food and Drug Administration (FDA). They are not all bad, but some people are particularly sensitive to them, and they can adversely affect hyperactive children.

In order to test your own sensitivity, or that of your child, to certain additives, you need to begin a very restricted diet of bland basic foods. Gradually reintroduce one at a time those foods that are suspect and record any reactions. It is best to consult a nutritionist, naturopath, or doctor who specializes in food sensitivities when conducting a test such as this.

The best advice for planning good nutrition is to avoid foods that you know you are allergic to and to maintain a balanced diet. Eat low-fat, high-fiber, naturally sweetened foods, and let moderation and common sense be your guide.

Calorie Chart

The word *calorie* refers to a unit of energy. Calories represent the amount of energy needed to burn a particular substance. The number of calories each person needs for maximum energy depends on age, sex, occupation, and lifestyle. The following chart serves as a guide for the amount of daily caloric intake for various groups of people:

MEN

Age	Lifestyle	Calories Needed Daily
18–35	Inactive	2,500
	Active	3,000
	Very active	3,500
36–70	Inactive	2,400
	Active	2,800
	Very active	3,400

WOMEN

Age	Lifestyle	Calories Needed Daily
18–55	Inactive	1,900
	Active	2,100
	Very active	2,500
56–70	Inactive	1,700
	Active	2,000

In their quest for health, fitness, and the perfect body, many people become almost obsessive about counting calories. Remember that it is not so much the number of calories you consume, but where they come from, that is important. In other words, it is better to eat 400 calories' worth of pasta and vegetables than of ice cream. The key to planning and following a healthy diet is balance. Eat a variety of whole foods from the basic food groups, and eliminate or moderate your consumption of those foods that you know are not good for you.

Orthomolecular Medicine

Ortho is the Greek word meaning "to correct." Two-time Nobel prize winner Linus Pauling coined the term *orthomolecular medicine* in 1968 to refer to a system of correcting the body's metabolism with the right combination of nutrients, such as vitamins, minerals, amino acids, and enzymes. All of these nutrients occur naturally in the body as a defense against illness, but sometimes the body becomes deficient in one or many of them.

In 1943, the National Resource Council's Food and Nutrition Board established the Recommended Dietary Allowances (RDAs) of various nutrients. In 1963, the Food and Drug Administration created minimum daily requirements called U.S. RDAs, which are used by food manufacturers. The levels of U.S. RDAs are based on the lowest levels necessary to prevent known diseases, such as scurvy, which are caused by deficiencies. However, these levels are not necessarily high enough to promote health and combat other common illnesses. Orthomolecular doctors and other scientists advocate setting nutritional standards not based on avoiding diseases, such as scurvy, but on promoting optimum health.

Orthomolecular medicine is holistic in that it considers mental and physical causes of biochemical imbalances in the body. Practitioners perform blood tests and use vitamin and mineral profiles to delineate levels for sixteen vitamins and thirty minerals. Many physical and mental disorders can be treated simply by supplementing deficiencies in these nutrients.

Since each individual is unique, each has different nutritional needs. People who take megadoses of nutrients should take breaks from their dosages in order to prevent overdose. Orthomolecular treatments should be supervised by a trained doctor or nutritionist.

EXERCISE

Most of us live rather sedentary lives—we drive instead of walking or riding a bike; we sit at work; and we watch television while resting on the couch. Yet exercise is vital to our physical and emotional health. It improves muscle tone and posture, increases strength and stamina, and can improve circulation and respiration. Not only does exercise reduce blood-fat levels, it can change large blood-fat globules (low-density lipoproteins) to smaller, less sticky ones (high-density lipoproteins) that move more easily and are less likely to clog arteries. Exercise also is good for the mind. It invigorates and energizes, and helps to relieve tension and anxiety. By helping to release substances that affect emotions, such as adrenaline and noradrenaline, exercise can even relieve the symptoms of depression. Have you ever heard of a runner's high? The explanation for runners' "addiction" to their exercise is that it helps to release endorphins and enkephalins, which have a mood-elevating effect. When you exercise, your body gets in shape and your mind begins to relax.

There are several different kinds of exercise, and a good workout routine should include a little of each. *Isotonic* exercises, such as weight training, stretching, and yoga, develop muscle strength and flexibility. They do not have the aerobic benefits of improving respiration and circulation, but they are essential for toning slack muscles and building strength. *Stretching* exercises, as part of your warmup and cool-down, are a must in any kind of workout.

Aerobics refer to sustained exercise that increases the amount of oxygenated blood carried to muscles and organs. In other words, any activity that increases your breathing and heart rate is aerobic: aerobic dance, step aerobics, running, jogging, fitness walking, cycling, swimming, and cross-country skiing. Stationary bicycles, Life-cycles, and StairMasters are aerobic fitness machines. When you perform an aerobic exercise, you should maintain your training-level heart rate for fifteen minutes or longer in order to receive maximum results. (See the chart on p. 68.) Aerobic exercise improves the respiratory and circulatory systems. It strengthens the heart muscle, makes arteries and veins more elastic, and lowers blood-fat and body-fat levels.

Anaerobic exercise is the opposite of aerobic exercise. It is characterized by short bursts of energy, such as sprinting. Although anaerobic exercise does develop muscle strength, it does not improve circulation and respiration.

When you plan an exercise regimen, consider activities that you enjoy, that are feasible, and that you will want to do. That way you'll have a better chance of maintaining your exercise routine. Some people like to exercise alone —it is "quiet" time to think or clear the mind. Others prefer to exercise with a partner or a group because other people can be a good source of motivation and can make exercise a fun social event. You also need to consider how much time you can allot to the activity. When you have a very busy schedule, it is easy to forgo the exercising, especially if you are tired. Just try to remember that the more you exercise, the more energy you will have in the long run for all of your life's activities.

If you are over the age of forty and have been relatively inactive, are pregnant, or have another medical condition, you should consult a physician and have a complete physical exam before beginning an exercise program. When you start, begin slowly and gradually increase the duration and intensity of your workouts. Warming up is a must—stretch your muscles slowly and smoothly for at least five minutes. The endurance phase of your workout should last approximately twenty to thirty minutes, getting your pulse rate up to training level. Cooling down is also imperative—spend five to ten minutes walking briskly and doing more stretching exercises.

The following chart will help you determine your training-level pulse rate. The resting pulse of adults is generally sixty to eighty beats per minute. To take your pulse, use the first three fingers of your hand to feel the beat in your temple or neck. Count the number of beats in fifteen seconds and multiply that by four to equal one minute.

Age	Beats per minute for Training Level
20	138–158
25	137–156
30	135–154
35	134–153
40	132–151
45	131–150
50	129–147
55	127–146
60	126–144
65	125–142
70	123–141
75	122–139
80	120–138
85	119–136

Once you get into the swing of an exercise routine, you'll probably look forward to the activities—and even feel bad if you skip a session. Remember to use common sense when you are exercising, especially if you do strenuous aerobic activity. Here are some tips:

• Do not exercise if you are ill, dizzy, or feel faint. If any of these feelings occur during a workout, cool down by walking and stretching, and then take off a day or two.

- Do not exercise if you feel severe muscle or joint pain; take a few days off and begin again gradually. If pain persists, consult a physician.
- Always warm up and cool down to avoid stiff or injured muscles.
- Allow two hours after meals before exercising.
- Avoid exercising in very hot weather and dress warmly in cold weather if you exercise outside; even if you perspire, keep all of your clothing on to avoid chilled muscles that can result in cramps or pulls.
- "No pain, no gain" may be true to a degree, but you should build the intensity of your workout gradually. Use common sense, listen to your body and mind, and don't overdo it!

CHAPTER THREE

Maintaining Health

If you're like most Americans, you've been taught to overlook the body unless sickness flairs up. You don't concern yourself with developing skills to promote better health because you've been guided by a health-care system that unfortunately lacks a preventive component. In this country, great attention is devoted to complex disease-care technology, but little regard is paid to health maintenance.

Such an approach, besides being costly, creates an indifference to effective resources for prevention. American medicine overlooks a machine so complicated and intricate that a team of scientists from around the world could not have dreamed it up—the human body. The self-regulating properties of the body are interrelated and complex—the body is at once scout, chemist, physician, construction worker, nutritionist, and manager. Derived from two cells, the body is made of about one hundred trillion cells that vary enormously in function, size, and shape. Five types of tissue, each of which is dependent on the others, are found in the body—blood, nerve, muscle, epithelial (skin) and connective tissue. Two extensive communication systems facilitate the body's coordination of its hundreds of muscles and bones and enhance orchestration of myriad functions. A network of cables called the nervous system relays messages to and from all parts of the body. And the endocrine system triggers the release of chemical messengers called hormones into the bloodstream to be transported to certain organs to regulate activities. Together, these hormones, nerves, and the brain, the master-control center, form an elaborate organization that is interrelated to a degree that was not dreamed of even a few decades ago. This organization enables the body to conduct thousands of simultaneous jobs without interruption, and to replace weak cells with exact replicas so as not to interfere with any process.

This scheme within the body also allows us to maintain good health. The body's interrelated systems fight disease and invasion, counteract nutritional deficiencies, and combat stress. Should a malfunction occur in the body, for example, a coordinated effort is immediately launched to promote healing. When we receive a wound, the circulatory system immediately transports legions of the body's immune system to close the wound and fight invading bacteria.

Constant communication among systems enables the body to fight off nutritional deficiencies. The body constantly measures its nutrient levels and can signal the small intestine to take in additional nutrients from foods when supplies are low. If we have consumed too much of nutrient-rich foods, the body will send a message to release most of that nutrient from the body. This sensitive meter can be thrown off, however, when we take in immense amounts of nutrients from some food sources and vitamin supplements, with the result that the body retains excessive and sometimes toxic nutrient levels.

Another natural mechanism is activated when we bask in the sun and the body utilizes the sun's ultraviolet rays to synthesize amounts of vitamin D. When vitamin D levels are nearly satisfied, the body will automatically shut off its production. However, if foods or vitamin supplements of vitamin D are ingested, the body retains any excessive levels in the liver and body fat. Consequently, very high doses of vitamin D can have unhealthy side effects.

Besides maintaining a nutritional balance, the body often takes the lead in promoting health. For example, when we regularly practice relaxation techniques such as meditation, yoga, or breathing, our body begins to adapt to the more relaxed state. Soon, the body will require greater and greater amounts of the adrenal hormones before it will launch a stress response.

If we set the stage for better health, then, the body, in an effort to maintain equilibrium and prevent overwork, will follow our lead. In order for its self-regulating properties to take effect, however, we must supply it with the basic tools of prevention. Good nutrition, exercise, emotional support and a feeling of well-being will not only enhance our health, but our day to-day living. While allopathic prescription drugs and surgery are certainly valuable life-saving techniques, it is our lifestyle that dictates whether we will even take the drugs, what happens after hospitalization, and what we will do to promote recovery. What is too often missing from allopathic medicine is *us*.

Natural therapies, in contrast, are gentle and safe enough to become part of our day-to-day lives. In addition, exercise, good nutrition, homeopathy, and meditation promote our health while preventing disease. In short, natural therapies are *simultaneously preventive and therapeutic*.

ACUPRESSURE

While mysterious and enigmatic to the West, this traditional medicine has served China for centuries as a very effective therapy. As you learned in Chapter Two, the emphasis is on maintaining health, but illness can arise when energy in any of the fourteen meridians in the body becomes blocked, misdirected, reversed, or stagnant.

Acupressure treatment involves a variety of point-stimulation techniques that redirect the flow of energy in the body, and, in the process, prompt secretion of the body's most potent painkillers: endorphins and enkephalins. It's worth noting here that lifestyle factors such as good nutrition, adequate sleep, exercise, and relaxation are all necessary for the body to respond optimally to acupressure and other meridian therapies. You may be surprised to learn that you can administer therapy in one part of the body that is distant from the inflamed or affected area; by stimulating points on the feet, for example, you can relieve menstrual pain and breast tenderness. This is possible because these three areas are linked by the liver channel, which traverses the area of the body from the big toe of each foot to a point below the breast. In addition to using points on the fourteen meridians, you can also access any organ-energetic system through points on any of the three primary microsystems found in the ears, feet and hands; a complete microcosm of the body's energetic framework is found there.

When used safely, acupressure is a gentle treatment that can be performed almost anywhere and at any time. However, it should never be used as a *primary* treatment to relieve excessive bleeding, vaginal discharges, or undiagnosed pain, each of which can be an indication of serious illness requiring prompt medical care. Similarly, acupressure should *not* replace standard medical care for cancer or any kind of infection, and should be used during pregnancy only for specific ailments (see Chapter Six), because it may promote abortion or premature labor.

With practice, you can learn to apply acupressure quite effectively. Apply this therapy twice daily to alleviate gynecological symptoms such as those associated with menopause and menstruation. For chronic conditions like osteo-arthritis, acupressure can be used every day or more frequently if pain intensifies. Following is a description of various acupressure remedies for stimulating the immune system and promoting relaxation. Once you become skilled at obtaining relief through acupressure, you can maximize health by maintaining restored energy balance. Applying the points discussed here will increase overall vitality and stimulate energy flow. In addition, practices like tai chi chuan, when used over the long term, can be quite helpful in bolstering health and vitality.

Applying Acupressure

Before you begin, some preparation is necessary. Wear loose, comfortable clothing while you lie down or sit in a relaxed position. You can either treat yourself, or ask a friend to treat you by following the instructions below. First, become familiar with the acupressure points. Once you have read about them here, consult the illustrations at the back of the book, and identify the location of each point on your body. With your fingers, feel for a slight depression underneath the skin; this is the point. You may also know it by a strange tingling sensation, or even soreness that occurs to the touch.

Acupressure treatment is effective because you are stimulating meridian points that are like wells where the energy of the body bubbles up to the surface and is accessible to treatment by needles, magnets, or touch. Therefore, extreme pressure is not necessary nor beneficial. You can achieve several different effects on your *chi* by applying different types of pulsing techniques to the point, either to strengthen, diminish, or relax *chi*. There are usually several points that can provide relief for a condition, and some of these points will work better for you than others.

Acupressure is most effective when several points, as opposed to a single point, are part of your treatment plan. In general, self-help acupressure is good for symptomatic relief of conditions like headaches and cramps. To increase the benefits available through meridian therapy, consult a qualified acupuncturist who can assess the underlying energetic imbalance that is resulting in the symptoms causing you discomfort, and who can then administer appropriate treatments to resolve the imbalance and prevent recurrence of the symptoms.

Strengthen the flow of *chi* by applying pressure to a point. Use the fatty portion of your fingertip to bear down on the point for two to three minutes. For beginners, this is the best way to ensure making contact with the point. Pressure should be heavy enough to create a sensation, but not so heavy that it causes you to flinch or tense up. Once you become proficient at applying acupressure, you'll be able to produce intense stimulation with even slight pressure, so you can use only your fingertip to manipulate the points. To disperse energy flow, use the fatty portion of your fingertip to make a steady, circular motion around the point for two to three minutes. Be sure to apply pressure. To relax *chi*, simply rest the palm of the hand on the point, or stroke it gently with your fingers for several minutes.

While you are applying acupressure, it's important to visualize the *chi* flowing through your body to the affected areas. You can augment your healing energy by visualizing that universal *chi* with its restorative powers is also entering your body. Once you have succeeded in unblocking a point, you should feel the tension diminish beneath your fingers, and a slight pulse return. Releasing a point is often like peeling an onion. As the layers of tension are released, you can apply increasing amounts of pressure to the point to release it further.

The following points are useful for relaxation and for

strengthening the immune system. Unless otherwise noted, press points firmly for two to three minutes.

Reduce Stress, Anxiety, and Tension.   Anxiety may result from an imbalance in the energetics of any of the yin organs: heart, liver, spleen, kidney, or pericardium, and treatment is aimed at restoring balance to the energetic orb involved.

- *Yintang:* You'll find this point between the eyebrows, above the nose.
- *Stomach 36:* This point is located on the calf, four finger-widths below the bottom of the kneecap, one finger-width outside the shinbone. The point is on a muscle, which you can feel move if you flex your foot.
- *Heart 7:* This point is on the outer side of the forearm at the upper crease of the wrist.
- *Pericardium 6:* You can locate this point about three finger-widths from the upper crease of the wrist on the inner forearm, the point between the two tendons.

Strengthen the Immune System.   The *wei chi,* or "defensive *chi,*" flows at the surface of the body and protects us from invasion by exterior "pernicious" influences such as wind, heat, cold, dampness, summer heat, or dryness. The body's defenses can also become compromised when we indulge excessively in standing, sitting, lying down, physical feats, or overusage of the eyes. Treatment involves lifestyle changes, as well as strengthening energy flow to the internal organs.

- *Stomach 36:* This point is located on the calf, four finger-widths below the bottom of the kneecap, one finger-width outside the shinbone. The point is on a muscle, which you can feel move if you flex your foot.

* *Large intestine 4:* You'll feel this acupressure point on the upper part of the web between the thumb and forefinger on the back of the hand.

* *Large intestine 11:* When the elbow is flexed (bent) and the palm is facing down, this point is in the depression at the outer end of the elbow crease.

* *Gallbladder 39:* This point is situated about four finger-widths above the outer ankle bone, between the back edge of the fibula and the tendons that run there.

Increase Vitality.   Having an abundance of energy and a zest for life is a result of both a balanced *chi* and a healthy lifestyle. Pressing these points for two to three minutes will give your *chi* a boost, but the rest is up to you!

* *Stomach 36:* This point is located on the calf, four finger-widths below the bottom of the kneecap, one finger-width outside the shinbone. The point is on a muscle, so you'll know you're in the right place if you can feel it move when you flex your foot.

* *Governing vessel 4:* This point is situated on the spine, between the second and third lumbar vertebrae, at about the same level as the waist.

* *Conception vessel 4:* This point is located four finger-widths directly below the bellybutton, or two thumb-widths above the top of the pubic bone.

ACUPUNCTURE

An ancient meridian therapy like acupressure, acupuncture has weathered the test of time in China as a requisite treatment. It was not until the 1970s, when a cultural exchange was nurtured between China and the United States, that many Americans discovered that the vitality and restorative powers of acupuncture were the best-kept secret of the East.

As you learned in Chapter Two, acupuncture is based on the same principles as acupressure. The great strength of acupuncture is that energetic imbalances can be detected and adjusted by a well-trained therapist *before* they manifest as physical symptoms. In fact, the tenet of prevention is so strong in Eastern medicine that payment to early doctors was made only for *well* patients. The superior doctors prevented illness, while the less skilled doctors treated illness! And, while the emphasis is on prevention, energy imbalance that occurs in any of the body's meridians can result in illness.

Unlike acupressure, which can be self-applied, acupuncture must be performed by a skilled professional. (See Chapter Two for tips on choosing an acupuncturist.) An acupuncturist will diagnose the source of a specific energy problem, a complicated task requiring years of training and clinical experience—keep in mind that, in traditional Chinese medicine, no two people have the same illness or even energy pattern! In Western medicine, a headache is generally treated only as a headache. However, in Chinese medicine each disease can be identified as having many causes. An acupuncturist will want to know where the headache occurs and under what circumstances so that the meridian(s) involved may be identified and treated. Like all natural healers, an acupuncturist is concerned with all aspects of your health, so expect to spend at least thirty minutes discussing your symptoms, feelings, and lifestyle. He or she will probe into the possible reasons for *chi* to become imbalanced, which include poor nutrition, lack of exercise, emotional stress, fatigue, bad posture, compromised breathing, and pollution or physical growths such as tumors or scar tissue. An acupuncturist will notice many symptoms of altered energy that you and I might take for granted—like the hue of your complexion, the condition of your nails, your pulse rate, the sound of your voice, even your body odor—all of which offer clues to the nature of your constitution as well as to any underlying energy imbalances. The acupuncturist will take your pulse on many levels, and also examine your tongue—its shape, color, and any coating—for telltale signs of imbalance.

Once your imbalance or illness is diagnosed, your acupuncturist may recommend a treatment that may include any number of lifestyle changes, as well as setting up a session for acupuncture therapy. Acupuncture treatment involves a variety of needling techniques that redirect the flow of energy, and, in the process, relieve symptoms of pain by prompting secretion of the body's painkilling endorphins and enkephalins. Your therapist can manipulate your *chi* from any of the 365 primary points on the body, as well as many "extra points." Each of these points have particular effects on the *chi*, and various techniques may be applied to each point in order to activate energy or disperse it. Stimulating points like those used in acupressure treatment (discussed previously), he or she may administer therapy in one part of the body that is distant from the inflamed or affected area; stimulating points on the feet, for example, can relieve menstrual pain and breast tenderness. This is possible because these three areas are linked by the liver channel, which spans most of the body. So don't be surprised if your therapist accesses your menstrual pain, for example, through points on the ears, feet, or hands. The systems of the ear, foot, and hand acupuncture each contain a microcosm of the body's energetic framework!

To achieve certain effects, your therapist may use a variety of painless techniques, including lifting, thrusting, rotating, and vibrating the needles. How far a needle is inserted depends on the location of the point and the sensation you feel, but generally ranges from one-half inch to one inch. There are many techniques used for manipulating needles, depending upon the style of acupuncture in which the therapist has been trained. There is not just one style of acupuncture! Needle technique varies, for example, among Chinese, Japanese, and Korean styles of acupuncture. Some styles require significant needle manipulation and strong *chi* sensation, while others use different approaches to yield the same effects. In some techniques the needles are quickly inserted and removed, and in others they are left in the skin for up to thirty minutes and rotated occasionally.

When acupuncture needles are inserted, you may feel any number of sensations: tingling, a "rush" of sensation that radiates into the surrounding area, slight pain, warmth that radiates to the surrounding area, heaviness, or numbness. If you feel nothing, it usually means that your therapist hasn't contacted the *chi* yet. He or she will probably twist the needle or reinsert it until successful. The process of manipulating the needle until there is some sensation is called "getting the *chi*." It should be noted, however, that some very effective styles of acupuncture—Japanese, for example—use very little stimulation.

Although you may feel a slight pain when the point is inserted, the pain should subside when pushed deeper. But don't worry, a skilled acupuncturist has perfected a lightning-fast but gentle insertion technique. In fact, before learning their craft, acupuncture students must first master insertion of these extremely fine needles through dozens of layers of paper without bending them even slightly.

Your acupuncturist may also use *moxibustion,* burning of dried or ground leaves of the moxa plant (Artemisia vulgaris), called "Moxa-wool," to stimulate an acupuncture point. In general, needling of points moves and regulates the *chi* of the body. Moxa, when warm, has the property of being able to *tonify,* or add *chi* to the body, as well as to remove obstructions within the channels. Therefore, if a disharmony is a result of cold or deficiency (for example, menstrual cramps that subside with heat and pressure, making you want to curl up in bed with a heating pad), moxibustion would be recommended. There are two main techniques: For direct moxibustion, your acupuncturist will place a pile of Moxa-wool on a slice of ginger or garlic directly on the point and light it. For indirect moxibustion, she or he will burn a stick of moxa leaves near the acupuncture point until it is warm. Similarly, the tip of an inserted acupuncture needle can be warmed to increase stimulation. This technique is more of a yang, or warm, technique than needling.

Once your session is finished, or even before, you may notice instant relief and a feeling of overall well-being. Often changes begin to be noticed most dramatically between treatments. Once you have restored vitality and energy, exercises like tai chi chuan or meditation can be used over the long term to bolster health and prevent recurrence.

Like acupressure, acupuncture is a gentle, effective treatment when used properly. However, some precautions should be taken. Never use acupuncture as a *primary* treatment to relieve excessive bleeding, vaginal discharges, or undiagnosed pain, each of which can be an indication of serious illness requiring prompt medical care. Consult a physician first to rule out serious illness. Similarly, acupuncture should *not* replace standard medical care for cancer or any kind of serious infection or illness. Acupuncture is safe during pregnancy when administered by appropriately trained and licensed acupuncturists. There are a number of points forbidden during pregnancy, and some acupuncturists wait until the second trimester to provide treatment; however, acupuncture treatment is safe and effective for treating complaints throughout pregnancy including morning sickness, abdominal pain, edema, vaginal spotting, low-back pain and frequent urination. Acupuncture treatments during pregnancy should be used in conjunction with care by a medical doctor or a certified nurse-midwife and are never a substitute for regular prenatal medical care.

If the above precautions are heeded, there is no danger that acupuncture will make any conditions worse or interfere with drug treatment for diabetes, heart disease, epilepsy or hypertension (high blood pressure). Multiple acupuncture treatments may even reduce the need for drugs to lower blood sugar or blood pressure, or drugs to control seizures. Do *not,* however, eliminate any of these medications except under the supervision of your physician.

AEROBIC EXERCISE

Aerobic exercise can be a virtual panacea for many complaints, from menstruation to menopause. When performed regularly, or at least four times each week for at least twenty minutes, but preferably for forty minutes, aerobic exercise *does* seem to work miracles. Besides treating discomfort stemming from gynecological and other women's health problems, aerobic exercise has many preventive benefits as well. It lowers risk of heart disease by decreasing blood pressure and increasing the "good" HDL cholesterol that prevents the "bad" LDL cholesterol from clogging the arteries. Aerobic exercise also improves circulation and fights the creeping pound syndrome that can occur during the middle years. An aerobic exercise regimen can also lower blood sugar, making it useful for diabetics, and it can prevent osteoporosis.

With so many benefits, launching an aerobic exercise program may be the best decision you ever made! If you've never exercised before, or if it has been at least several months since you've worked out, it's best to start with a walking program and gradually increase the intensity of your workout.

Walking

Even walking at a leisurely pace of three miles per hour, five times per week, provides wonderful health benefits. This routine lowers cardiovascular risk by raising the "good" HDL cholesterol. However, this pace does not provide the aerobic benefits that are more effective in protecting our hearts, and relieving hormone-related discomforts during menstruation and menopause, so let that incentive help you to increase your pace. Exercising regularly so that your heart rate is within appropriate training levels (see "Exercise," Chapter Two), will also help you to tone muscles, lose fat, and possibly shed body weight (muscles weigh slightly more than fat).

Before embarking on a walking program, you should invest in a good pair of athletic shoes. Because a walker strikes the ground heel-first, then pushes off with the toes, walking shoes should have a firm heel counter (the cup around the heel), a flexible forefoot that bends easily at the ball of the foot, and longitudinal stability. To make sure the shoe is stable enough, try to twist it; an adequately rigid shoe will not give in.

Start at a moderate stride, and soon you will settle into your own pace. Whatever your gait, be consistent. Exercise during a time of the day when it is most enjoyable—after a long day's work when the mind needs a rest, or early in the morning when you're most energetic. If you walk on a track or other enclosed area, take a Walkman and listen to an audiobook or your favorite tape. The most important thing is to enjoy yourself!

Running

Once you feel confident and comfortable with a walking regimen, or if you have been working out regularly at another activity, you may want to progress to running. The best transition to running is a walk-run, walk-run sequence. Gradually increase the running component. When you run, be sure to go at your own pace, and if you run in a gymnasium or popular fitness area, resist the temptation to speed up as others pass you, or you will tire prematurely.

During your workout, it is best to learn to focus your mind on other things besides the distance you have run, and have yet to go. Focusing on your task can sometimes seem to make each foot drag and every step require extra effort, especially on days when you feel somewhat tired. Some runners develop adaptive ways of meditating while running. For example, you may have thoughts of being tired or bored, but not allow them to interfere with your performance by slowing down or quitting. Practicing meditation at home can be helpful in this endeavor. When you finish a run, you will feel energized, stimulated (from the painkilling endorphins and enkephalins), and completely relaxed. A good run can provide a wonderful transition from a nerve-racking day in the office to a smooth and energetic evening.

Just like walking, running requires the purchase of a good shoe. A running shoe is similar to a walking shoe but has a few more features to accommodate the greater impact that running imposes on the feet. A running shoe should be heavily cushioned under the heel and the ball of the foot—most runners land on one or both of these parts of the foot. The shoe should also have a roomy toe box so toes are not pinched when the foot is flexed, and a rigid heel counter to stabilize the foot. Shin splits, which is pain along the bone in the front of your calf, usually indicates that your shoes are ready for a trade-in because they do not provide adequate support or cushioning, but it can also mean that you are working too hard and should slow down the pace or cut back on mileage.

If you become an exercise enthusiast and take part in long workouts, you may need to increase potassium-rich foods in the diet, because heavy exercise tends to lower stores of potassium and salt in the body. Potassium-rich foods include oranges, tomatoes, potatoes, and bananas. Most of us consume enough salt in our diet to compensate for even a tough workout. However, if you crave salty food after a workout, especially on a very hot day, or long workout, it's okay to consume some salty foods at your next meal to satisfy your body's needs.

Before beginning any exercise program, consult your physician if you are more than forty years old, overweight, have diabetes, high blood pressure, cardiovascular disease, history of stroke, or any other serious condition.

AROMATHERAPY

Like herbalism, aromatherapy draws on the healing powers of plants. But unlike the botanical therapies that utilize parts of or the whole plant, aromatherapists use only the essential oils found in tiny glands throughout the plant. Chemicals in the oils are suspected to interact with each person's biochemistry to rejuvenate the body and the mind, and to heal a range of conditions from nausea to emotional upset. Oils can be either inhaled, or they can be applied directly to the body to permeate the skin.

Aromatherapy can be a strong stimulant to the mind and body because it utilizes the sense of smell, estimated to be ten thousand times stronger than any of the other four senses. Its powerful effect on the mind and body can be demonstrated as follows. Hold a pine cone or twigs of a fir tree in front of you and inhale. If you are an outdoors enthusiast, you will probably reexperience the cool, invigorating air of a summer vacation or retreat in the mountains. You may begin to breathe more fully and deeply, and your metabolism will slow as your mind envisions this haven of tranquility. Similar physiological and emotional effects can be promoted by essential oils. Because oils help to balance emotions, they tend to eradicate the cause of pain, tension, and diseases. Oils have other healing properties as well, from antiseptic to decongestant.

Because little research has been done in this area, scientists are not sure why aromatherapy works. They do know that essential oils are made up of as many as several hundred chemicals including alcohols, esters, ketones, phenols, and aldehydes. Alcohols and esters offer more gentle healing effects and are safer than high concentrations of ketones, phenols, and aldehydes. The latter group may have adverse effects, so should be used under the supervision of an aromatherapist. Just as scientists suspect that the many chemicals in herbs work synergistically to heal with minimal side effects, they believe that chemicals in essential oils work the same way. When isolated, the aldehyde called citral that is found in lemon oil, for example, becomes very toxic and can cause severe skin irritations. But when part of lemon's essential oil, citral contributes to its beneficial effects. Synthetic oils do not produce this natural synergy, one reason why they are not recommended by aromatherapists.

Like many natural healing techniques, aromatherapy has its root in ancient times. The Egyptians were the first to use balsamic substances to mummify their cats and kings. Records dating back five thousand years ago show that fragrant oils, scented barks and resins, spices and aromatic vinegars were used in medicine, embalmings, and religious ceremonies. Much later, the Greeks, most notably Hippocrates, advocated a daily aromatic cleansing and a fragrant massage to maintain health, a philosophy very much shared by today's aromatherapists. Aromatherapy is used worldwide today, especially in Europe, where aromatherapeutic remedies line the shelves of pharmacies. In France, essential oils are covered by national health insurance.

Essential oils can be purchased in your local health-food store or body shop in one-fourth-ounce or one-half-ounce brown-glass bottles. The cost of the half-ounce size ranges from $3 to $12. Prior to use as a remedy, concentrated essential oil should be diluted in a carrier oil or lotion to facilitate application. Cold-pressed vegetable oils that contain vitamins B and E are easily absorbed. Grapeseed, safflower, and sweet-almond oils are lighter than wheat-germ, olive, and avocado oils. The latter group may be mixed with lighter oil to moisturize dry skin. Skin that is oily, inflamed, or has acne, will benefit from the use of jojoba oil, which is not actually an oil but a wax. Carrier lotion, made from emulsified oil and water, is a good option if you prefer an application that is not greasy. Before using any mixture, apply a very small amount to your skin to test for a reaction.

Essential oil should be diluted in carrier lotion in the following proportions: four drops to two teaspoons, five drops to one-half fluid ounce, ten drops to one fluid ounce, twenty drops to two fluid ounces, and so on. Measure oil or lotion first, then add essential oil and shake. Keep bottles tightly sealed and in a dark, cool place to avoid heat, light, and air, all of which detract from its therapeutic powers. Distilled essential oils will keep for several years, but when mixed into cold-pressed vegetable oils, they should be used within six months. Other oil-based mixes will keep for nine months, and lotion-based mixes for at least one year.

When drawing a bath with essential oil, add six to ten drops to a full bathtub of water—the hotter the water, the faster the oils will dissolve and begin working. Oils won't dissolve if you drop the solution directly into the bathwater, however. Blend oils with a carrier oil (see the previous dilutions), and sprinkle the solution in the bathtub.

Learning about essential oils can be quite gratifying. Testing a variety of remedies, each of which responds differently to your body chemistry, will enable you to develop an individual and effective treatment. Like any natural therapy, you could learn a great deal by seeking the advice of a professional. (To find an aromatherapist in your area, consult the National Association for Holistic Aromatherapy listed in the back of the book.)

If you decide to treat yourself, be sure to follow the instructions carefully. Aromatherapy may be performed on a weekly basis, or whenever specific symptoms arise. In future chapters, we will discuss therapeutic applications for specific conditions from menstrual problems to menopause. Unless otherwise noted, you should notice results right away, and do not need to continue therapy after your condition is improved. Aromatherapy may be used in conjunction with most natural therapies, but may interfere with the effectiveness of herbs and homeopathy.

One precaution is that you use essential oils only under the advice of a professional aromatherapist if you have high blood pressure, epilepsy, or any nerve disorder. Some essential oils may adversely affect these conditions.

Following are suggested solutions for promoting relaxation and increasing vitality:

- Lavender, sandalwood, melissa (lemon balm), chamomile, clary sage, geranium, and rose are all soothing to the emotions. A mixture of melissa and clary sage will uplift you on even the most trying days. For rapid relief of headaches and/or irritability, sprinkle two drops each of melissa, chamomile, and lavender onto a tissue and inhale deeply.

- Add three drops of lavender and two drops of rose to carrier oil and add to your bath to encourage relaxation.

- Use the following massage mix for overall balancing and relaxing: four drops each of lavender and clary sage, two drops of rose or melissa to one fluid ounce of carrier oil or lotion. Apply to the shoulders. Then use a kneading motion of the fingers to apply pressure to the shoulders and the periphery. You will relieve knots of tension there, which should have an overall effect of relaxation.

BREATHING FOR RELAXATION

Stress and the Mind-Body Link

Stress has been recognized as an increased risk for heart attack and other diseases, as well as an important influence on our experience of symptoms and illness. Many women's health conditions are thought to have a psychosocial component; for example, women who are depressed or anxious may find that symptoms of bodily discomfort are intensified. Research on the frontier of mind-body medicine currently explores the role that certain emotions and psychosocial factors may play in illness. However, it has been long established that physiological changes associated with chronic or prolonged stress can have harmful effects on the body. Stress can contribute to elevated blood pressure, increased susceptibility to infections, some stomach and intestinal disorders, and chronic fatigue syndrome. Stress can also become manifested in parts of the body, causing muscle and joint problems. Conversely, our experience of illness or any unpleasant symptoms can be transformed by mind-body relaxation techniques such as biofeedback (Chapter Two), hatha-yoga, hypnosis (Chapter Eight) or meditation. Symptoms of even severe pain, when lulled by inner tranquility, can become tolerable and sometimes eliminated.

Our physiological experience of stress is called the "fight or flight" response. The body reacts to stresses of any kind, whether physical or emotional, actual or imagined, life-threatening or trivial, with a cascade of metabolic changes. First, the brain causes the hormones adrenaline and noradrenaline to be released. These, in turn, fire off increases in heart rate, metabolism, blood pressure, breathing rate, and muscle tension. This is the body's way of gearing up for dramatic physical feats that, in the context of most of our lives, is usually unnecessary. If this peak metabolic state is prolonged, it can promote the body's disrepair and, subsequently, illness.

Alleviating the source of stress seems to be the most obvious and direct solution. Realistically, however, this is not always possible, nor even recommended on short notice. For example, quitting your job or breaking off an interpersonal relationship are major changes that often warrant time spent in much introspection and thought, possibly with the help of a good psychotherapist (see Psychotherapy, Chapter Two). On the other hand, if your frustrations are relatively minor, like those stemming from a daily traffic jam, incorporating simple relaxation exercises into your life may be all that is necessary to bring your mind and body back to a harmonious relationship. In either case, you can benefit immensely by learning relaxation techniques. Study results indicate that stress-reduction strategies, when practiced regularly, can raise the threshold of provocation before a stress response. In other words, not only can you learn to be calm in a stressful storm, but eventually it may take a sinking ship for anxiety to take its hold on you!

Changes in breathing quality are one of the first and most obvious signs that the body is launching a stress response. By interrupting the rapid breathing response, we can slow or even avert the stress response and those harmful metabolic changes. Breathing calms us, thus slowing our physical and emotional "fight or flight" reaction.

Breathing Healthfully

Healthy, relaxed breathing is abdominal, "belly," breathing. Abdominal breathing allows ten times more volume of air into the lungs than our typical chest breathing! This enormous increase in air supply allows much more oxygen to get into the bloodstream, so the heart can work more efficiently. Since more oxygen circulates in the bloodstream, the cells are better nourished and the blood supply does not have to be pumped as rapidly to deliver nutrients to the cells. Thus, the heart can slow down. This is, in fact, how we each breathed when we were born. Ironically, many people have unlearned natural, healthy breathing. They breathe every day in an accelerated fashion, rapid and shallow, just as if the body were responding to an emergency! Rapid and shallow breathing from the chest has the reverse effect of relaxed breathing: it causes poor oxygen delivery to the cells and consequently causes the heart to work harder. It triggers the body to step up other metabolic functions to prepare for strenuous physical and emotional exertion.

A good way to determine if you are "belly" breathing is to sit in a chair with your back straight and put one hand over your chest and another over your belly. Breathe in and watch your hands to see which one moves. Practice belly breathing by inhaling deeply while letting your belly go. It is the natural way to breathe, so once you relax, your body will let it happen. Once you become aware of your breathing patterns, you will be able to recognize the body's "fight or flight" response immediately, perhaps even before you are psychologically aware of stress.

Belly-Breathing Practice

Sit in a chair with your back straight, and place your hands just below your rib cage with fingertips barely touching. Breathe in deeply, watching your belly expand and the fingertips of each hand move away from each other. Practice expanding your belly without the deep breaths by pushing your abdominal muscles outward until you can see your stomach expand. Now inhale slowly, straighten your posture and stretch your spine a little until you feel the air rise to the very top of your lungs. Practice both deep breathing and belly expansion at the same time. Take in a breath slowly to a count of six. With your belly expanded, hold for a count of two. Exhale gradually for a count of six. Do this four or five times. At first you might feel some dizziness because your body is unaccustomed to this slower breathing. If this happens, alternate deep, slow breaths with slightly faster breaths until equilibrium is restored.

Because relaxed breathing enhances the enjoyment of almost any activity and can be accomplished in almost any place, it is a quite useful therapy. It augments the effectiveness of many other relaxation therapies, and may be used in conjunction with aerobic exercise, biofeedback (Chapter Two), hatha-yoga, hypnosis (Chapter Eight), imagery, meditation, and psychotherapy (Chapter Two).

HATHA-YOGA

Both stunning physical feats and intense health benefits mark the ancient Indian practice of hatha-yoga, the positions of which were adapted from the lithe jungle cat. There are two broad areas of yoga. We will cover hatha-yoga, consisting of the asanas, or body postures, here, and meditative yoga in the section headed "Meditation" later in this chapter.

Yoga therapy is based on ancient Indian philosophy that five "sheaths" exist in life, made up of physical, mental, and spiritual energies and thought. Imbalance of these sheaths can result in two types of disorders. Contagious diseases and accidental injuries are believed to have a physical origin and are treated with allopathic medicine. Most other diseases, including degenerative illnesses and psychosomatic disorders, are believed to arise from strong feelings of like or dislike that obstruct the flow of positive energy from the most important "bliss" sheath to the remaining sheaths. Treatment involves the asanas, or positions, which are practiced to stimulate key pressure points of vital energy in the body. Because energy flow massages, tones, and improves the efficiency of the internal organs, asanas are also preventive.

While strengthening energy flow is the primary goal of hatha-yoga, regular practice is also a marvelous stress-fighter and a great resource for improving general health. Yoga practice evokes a host of physiological changes. Heart and breathing rates are slowed, blood pressure is reduced, and oxygen consumption is lowered. Stress and tension are released from the body, so psychological benefits, including reduced anxiety, hostility, and aggression, as well as improved self-esteem, may all be reaped from practicing even the simplest of yoga positions. If you've ever seen a true yoga master, you may have marveled at the gymnastic-like feats she or he accomplished with seemingly little effort. Such people usually have practiced yoga for many years, so don't attempt such agile maneuvers yourself! As your flexibility increases, you can include more advanced positions in your regimen.

Yoga may be useful in counteracting a variety of conditions, from stress to aging. Stress has been recognized as an increased risk for heart attack and other diseases, as well as an important influence on our experience of symptoms and illness. Many women's health problems involving menstruation or menopause are believed to be exacerbated by anxiety or depression. Because hatha-yoga is useful in minimizing stress, it can reduce the stress-related symptoms of such health problems and lower our risk of developing certain illnesses. Hatha-yoga promotes spinal flexibility, so it can counteract many effects of aging. But it has advanced applications as well: it is being pioneered in the United States as a therapy for severe pain management. In the quiet and relaxed state of yoga, a person learns to recognize and let go of anxious thoughts that can heighten sensations of pain (for example, what is going to happen to me? How can I possibly bear this?). Thus, the experience of pain becomes bearable.

Treatment involves practicing asanas throughout the month. For maximum effectiveness, first perform the belly-breathing practice (see "Breathing for Relaxation") and the practice meditation (see "Meditation"), then the sun-salutation exercise, which follows here. In future chapters, we will discuss therapeutic applications for specific conditions. Yoga may be used in conjunction with any other natural therapy. But specific positions that may be harmful to those with certain medical conditions (noted in individual chapters) should be avoided.

Salutation to the Sun

In India, the "sun salutation" is performed by millions of people as a greeting to the day. It is a gentle but effective way to limber up the body and soothe the mind. You should warm up with this exercise before practicing remedies for individual conditions in successive chapters.

First, stand with back straight and palms together in front of you as if praying. Breathe deeply from your belly, and exhale several times. When you have centered yourself in the here and now, lean backward from your belly and head while raising the arms back and over the head. Hold this position for as long as possible without discomfort.

Then, drop your arms, torso, and head so that fingers touch the floor, bending from the abdomen. If you cannot touch the floor, drop as low as possible without bending the knees. Remain in this pose for a count of ten, or longer if you feel comfortable.

Kneel down by dropping the buttocks to the floor. Let your palms touch the floor, but keep the trunk of your body in an upright position. Hold this pose for a count of four.

Gently slide one leg behind you until it is fully extended, but continue to bend the other leg at the knee. Your weight should rest on your arms, which should be locked. Raise your head in a salute to the sun. Remain in this position for a count of six.

Slide your foot back into place, bending your knee. Let your knees drop to the floor, resting the buttocks on the heels of your feet. Then let your chest, then arms, neck, and head slowly sink down until your chest rests on your knees and your head is flat on the floor. Your arms are extended in front of you. Relax in this pose until you feel centered again, perhaps to a count of eight.

Gradually lift yourself up to a kneeling position again, with palms flat on the floor. Slide your leg behind you until it is fully extended, but continue to bend the other leg at the knee. Raise your head in a salute to the sun. Remain in this position for a count of six. Once you become more flexible through yoga practice, you can try a more advanced position. Slide both legs behind you until they are fully extended, resting most of your weight on your arms, which should be locked. Your feet should be flexed at the toes, and your entire body raised in the area by several inches. Your back should be arched and your head up. Hold this pose for a count of four, or until you tire. Release the pose by dropping your knees to the floor and unlocking your arms.

Bring in the knees and stand up. Once you have practiced yoga regularly, try getting up with a more advanced movement. Draw in the knees, and push your buttocks into the air as you straighten arms and legs. You will form a triangle with the floor. Hold this position for several counts, or as long as comfortable.

Now drop your arms, torso, and head so that fingers touch the floor, bending from the abdomen. If you cannot touch the floor, drop as low as possible without bending the knees. Remain in this pose for a count of ten, or longer if you feel comfortable.

Let your knees drop to the floor, resting the buttocks on the heels of your feet. Then let your chest, then arms, neck, and head slowly sink down until your chest rests on your knees and your head is flat on the floor. Your arms are extended in front of you. Relax in this pose until you feel centered again, perhaps to a count of eight.

Gently slide one leg behind you until it is fully extended, but continue to bend the other leg at the knee. Your weight should rest on your arms, which should be locked. Raise your head in a salute to the sun. Remain in this position for a count of six.

Let your knees drop to the floor, resting the buttocks on the heels of your feet. Next, let your chest, then arms, neck, and head slowly sink down until your chest rests on your knees and your head is flat on the floor. Your arms are extended in front of you. Relax in this pose to a count of eight.

Gradually lift yourself up to a kneeling position again, with palms flat on the floor. Then stand with your back straight and palms together in front of you as if praying. Breathe deeply with your belly and exhale several times. You are centered in the present.

Repeat this exercise using your other leg, then go out and enjoy the day!

HERBS

The soothing natural therapy of herbalism has been used by many ancient cultures to cure women's health problems. In recent years, healing herbs have gained favor with American women because they stimulate more gradual and gentler healing effects than their Western counterpart, prescription drugs. While the effects of the latter can often be equated with a club over the head, herbs restore the body and mind without overpowering either. In short, healing herbs revitalize at a pace and style that are instinctive to both the body and the mind.

Herbs act harmoniously in other ways as well. While the strength of a prescription drug lies in its active chemicals, herbs *become potent when activated by* the unique chemistry *between you and the herbs.* Each herb has its own feel and emphasis, and actuates a harmony with other herbs and with body sensations and emotions that are not discernible under a microscope. In another person, the same herb may have a different effect.

While based on some of the same principles as prescription drugs, herbal healing is nevertheless a very difficult therapy for us in the West to comprehend. How *does* one account for the fact that the same herb can promote the opposite effect when its dosage is altered? For example, the herb notoginseng, when given alone, will accelerate blood coagulation, but when combined with other herbs, it will do just the opposite. Or take schisandra fruit. When given in one dosage, it will stimulate the central nervous system; yet in a different amount, it will calm the system. Such phenomena are difficult to explain in Western scientific terms; of course, there is no need to do so if we accept herbal healing as an art.

Herbs, while gentler than drugs, contain small amounts of carcinogenic (cancer-causing) substances as well as amounts of cancer-fighting material called antioxidants. It was discovered in the 1980s that all plant substances, from mushrooms to bananas, contain minute amounts of these pro- and anticancer substances. Plants in themselves don't cause cancer because a balanced diet usually contains enough of both of these types of substances to have a neutralizing effect: no one eats mushrooms, a substance particularly high in carcinogenic material, in vast quantities at every meal, seven days a week. Like other plants, some healing herbs contain less and some more of these carcinogenic substances. You may want to avoid the latter herbs altogether (they are in each chapter) if you or anyone in your family has been diagnosed with some form of cancer.

While herbs can be self-applied (see below), you can learn more about the art of herbalism by making an appointment with an herbalist. If you were to visit an herbalist, she or he would likely treat you with a sophisticated mixture of herbs that act synergistically to complement your pattern of illness and health. An herbalist will sense the governing texture, or rhythm of your person, and match this to certain herbs, so that changes can take hold and grow.

A Chinese herbalist, of course, will treat you with a completely different criteria, based on a diagnosis using traditional Chinese-medicine principles, and provide you with herbs that are not generally available to the public. (For more information, see "Oriental Medicine," Chapter Two.)

If you decide to treat yourself, experimentation is recommended; some herbs will work better for you than others. Be sure to follow the instructions for herbal preparation, and pay special attention to any precautions. You should consult with a qualified professional, however, before undertaking any form of treatment. In addition, herbal therapy should never be used to substitute for standard medical care for any kind of serious illness or infection. Most of the herbs listed below and in subsequent chapters are available in dried form or in commercial teas at your local health-food store. Before going to purchase them, be sure to get to know your herbs and learn to identify their leaves, fruits, or bark. Rarely has there been a serious accident using healing herbs, but the handful of accidents reported involve using herbs that were incorrectly identified.

Taking the herbs below in the recommended quantities should produce results almost immediately. Once results are achieved, stop taking the herb. In all cases, do *not* take the herb longer or in greater doses than are recommended.

Healing herbs should not be taken while using aromatherapy or homeopathy, but can be combined with most other natural therapies.

Feverfew (*Matricaria* or *Chrysanthemum parthenium*). Most of the news that has been spread about the leaves of the feverfew plant, a member of the same family as the daisy and the dandelion, concerns its remarkable effectiveness in suppressing migraine headaches. But feverfew has many relaxing effects as well. Those with gynecological problems are the first to praise its antispasmodic effect, which causes the smooth muscles that line the uterine wall to relax. Feverfew is also believed to neutralize "bad" prostaglandins, the hormonelike chemicals in the body that are believed to play a role in causing menstrual cramps and in raising blood pressure. Because feverfew promotes complete relaxation, it may be very helpful on those high-stress days when it's hard to calm down.

Precautions: Feverfew may inhibit blood clotting, so people with clotting disorders or who are taking anticoagulants should not take it. The herb may also cause mouth sores or abdominal pain. If you experience these side effects, discontinue use immediately. Feverfew should not be used in larger amounts than listed below except under the supervision of a physician. Do not give this herb to children or elderly people. Pregnant women should avoid it.

Preparation: Add one-half to one teaspoonful per one cup of boiling water. Steep five to ten minutes. Drink up to two cups per day. Feverfew is available in commercial teas at your local health-food store.

Ginseng (*Panax quinquifolius* or *Panax ginseng*). The roots of the ginseng plant, a member of the ivy family, have attracted the attention of healers and peddlers alike for centuries. With sister plants native to both China and the United States, ginseng has been credited with enough properties to make it a cherished herb. It is rather difficult to grow, making it an expensive herb. However, ginseng's many preventive benefits are worth the price. The herb is believed to be an immune-system stimulant, although some studies have revealed contradictory results. This herb also has several wonderful benefits for improving health. Ginseng lowers levels of "bad" LDL cholesterol *and* raises amounts of "good" HDL cholesterol, which keeps the LDL cholesterol from clogging the arteries. Ginseng also has an anticlotting ability in the arteries, which reduces risk of heart disease and stroke. This herb may stimulate appetite because it lowers blood sugar, so watch out for possible creeping pounds! Because it lowers blood sugar, ginseng may be useful for diabetics. As a result of its proven effectiveness for many conditions, imitators and promoters claim that ginseng is in many products that unfortunately do not contain active amounts of the herb, so let the buyer beware.

Precautions: While generally safe, ginseng may increase blood pressure and produce cardiac arrhythmia, insomnia, allergies, or breast tenderness. Thus, those who are prone to or have any of these conditions should avoid using ginseng. Because of its anticlotting ability, ginseng should be avoided by hemophiliacs or others with blood-clotting problems. It also lowers blood sugar, so should be avoided by hypoglycemics. Do not give this herb to children or elderly people. Pregnant women should avoid it. Also, this herb may slightly increase levels of testosterone in some women. Thus, discontinue use if evidence of hormonal imbalance such as menstrual irregularities, premenstrual symptoms, or hair growth occurs while taking this herb.

Preparation: For a decoction, boil one-half teaspoonful of powdered root per cup of water for fifteen minutes. Take no more than three cups per day.

HOMEOPATHY

As you learned in Chapter Two, homeopathy treats "like with like"; that is, remedies are derived from substances that would stimulate the same symptoms in a healthy person. Gentle and completely safe remedies stimulate the body's natural defenses rather than inhibit or suppress the body's attempt to become well. Homeopathic treatments allow us to overcome the symptoms as well as the susceptibility that allowed the problem to develop in the first place. A person who has been treated homeopathically for many years is generally healthier and less prone to develop disease.

Part of homeopathy's allure is most likely its very individualized approach. Whether treatment is self-applied or given by a professional homeopath, one must have knowledge and awareness of symptoms and an individual's personality and idiosyncracies, which are then closely matched to a remedy. In fact, homeopathic healing will not be stimulated unless the characteristics of the remedy correspond quite well with the individual's symptoms. Conversely, if the wrong remedy is taken, no harmful effects will result; the treatment will simply have no effect.

If you were to visit a homeopath for a problem, your visit would involve lengthy discussion about your pattern of illness and health. A homeopath will delve into your likes and dislikes, habits, food cravings, emotional triggers, environmental stress, and your physical symptoms, to name a few. You might be asked questions like these: Are your feet often clammy and chilly? How are you affected by music? Do you push your feet out from under the blanket when you sleep? Do you have a tendency to reprimand? Do you have emotional fears or anxieties? Are you uncommonly tidy and clean, or disorderly? Is your pain found more on one side than another?

Like all holistic therapies, the treatment itself can be quite nurturing and may contribute to a greater capacity for self-healing. Even homeopathy founder Hahnemann rejected the current scientific dogma of his day, calling the action behind homeopathic medicine "almost purely spiritual." In Germany this therapy is commonly used in hospitals and private practice, and boasts a high success rate for curing a wide array of illnesses of both an acute and chronic nature.

Some homeopaths also have earned conventional allopathic medical degrees and so treat more serious and life-threatening illnesses with allopathic medicine. Chronic and mild illnesses are usually treated with the more gentle and sometimes slower action of homeopathic medicine. During diagnosis, a homeopathic medical doctor will likely have a good grasp of your unique symptoms of illness because she or he is also familiar with the natural "course" of a disease, and looks at the condition from a homeopathic perspective. This way, a suitable homeopathic remedy can be chosen for you.

Once a recommendation for a remedy is made, a homeopath will often discuss any suggestions for lifestyle changes with you, which may involve exercise, nutrition, posture, breathing, meditation, or psychotherapy. If a structural problem is interfering with a cure, a homeopath may send you to another professional for chiropractic or massage therapy. Of course, she or he will also give you a homeopathic remedy that closely matches your ailment and personality.

If you are treating yourself, it's important to match your feelings and physical symptoms as closely as possible with the remedies listed below, just as a homeopath would. Don't forget Hering's Law of Cure. Psychological symptoms often disappear first because homeopathy heals from the inside out. Symptoms should ideally dissipate from the top of the body to the bottom. Finally, symptoms should disappear in the reverse order that they appeared.

Remedies can be purchased in your local pharmacy or health-food store for a moderate cost. They are available in liquid form, which usually comes in small glass vials of solution with screw tops, in dried granules, or in pills that are impregnated with solution. The bottles are usually labeled by the number of serial dilutions, a higher potency having been diluted and vigorously shaken a greater number of times. For example, a 6c solution was diluted in a proportion of 1:100 and shaken, six times, and is not as potent as a 30c solution, which was put through the same process for a total of thirty times. Stored in a cool, dark place, homeopathic remedies should remain potent for up to several decades!

Unless otherwise noted, take a daily dose of 6c of the solutions listed below. For chronic conditions, a visit to a homeopathic physician is recommended. Stop taking medication once your ailment begins to improve. Remedies can be taken in between meals, or at least fifteen minutes after eating. If your medication has no effect, it usually indicates that you have taken the wrong remedy. In that case, review your symptoms, and, being as specific as possible, match them to another remedy.

Homeopathic solutions will not interfere with the action of prescription drugs. However, some drugs will block the effects of homeopathic remedies, at least to some degree. These include steroids, tranquilizers, birth control pills, sleeping pills, and antihistamines. Do *not* stop taking drugs prescribed by your physician without first consulting him or her. And, before taking any remedy, it is recommended to consult with an appropriate health professional. Homeopathy may be used in conjunction with acupuncture, chiropractic (Chapter Four), hypnosis (Chapter Eight), or psychotherapy (Chapter Two), but should not generally be used simultaneously with aromatherapy or herbs. The former's essential oils may inactivate the homeopathic remedy, as will coffee, alcohol, tobacco, perfumed cosmetics, and strong-smelling household cleansers.

For relaxation (to relieve stress, anxiety, insecurity), the following are recommended:

- *Phosphoric acid:* A gentle remedy for people who are usually lively and affectionate, highly strung, and sensitive, but become lethargic, irritable, and exhausted while under stress.
- *Picric acid:* When working late hours is the primary cause of stress, tension, and aggravation, this remedy can be very helpful.
- *Ignatia amara:* To soothe the pain of grief, humiliation, shock, or disappointment that is

accompanied by irritability or weepiness, try this
wonderful treatment.

• *Nux vomica:* This remedy is for the "workaholic" type,
whose stress and tension results from a frenetic lifestyle of too little sleep, a diet of rich foods, and little
or no exercise. Emotional symptoms are impatience,
anger, and contentiousness.

• *Lycopodium:* If you are jumpy and insecure about a
new job, a new relationship, or a performance like
giving a speech, and you dislike hot stuffy rooms and
crave sweets, this remedy can diminish your anxiety.

HYDROTHERAPY

Originally practiced in Germany and Austria by healer
priests in the last century, the natural, safe, and effective
therapy of hydrotherapy remains popular in spas and clinics. Based on the principle that treating one part of the
body will affect another or several parts, hydrotherapy
combines cryogenic (cold) and heat therapies with the
penetrating effects of water. Water treatment affects the
entire body, including the nervous system, the liver and its
chemistry, and the muscles. It improves oxygen delivery,
enhances digestion, and heightens skin sensations. You administer a form of hydrotherapy when you take a hot bath
to soothe tired, aching muscles. Pain is relieved when water therapy causes conversion of lactic acid in fatigued
muscles back into useful sources of energy.

To alleviate fatigue, try this invigorating, icy rubdown. It
will stimulate blood flow and revitalize the body. Dip a
towel sewn into the shape of a mitten into ice water, wring
out lightly and rub vigorously on the skin up and down two
or three times. Begin with the upper limbs. First rub the

fingers, then the arm all the way up to the shoulders. Dry each area and cover it before moving to the other arm. Apply this technique to the chest, the abdomen, the legs, the feet, then the back. Rub the skin until it is pink, harder if you can withstand it, especially on the arms and legs. This treatment enhances nerve and muscle tone and skin sensation, increases oxygen delivery to the tissues, and improves overall energy.

Another technique for invigorating body and mind is alternating a hot shower with a cold one.

IMAGERY

Popular since the thirteenth century, the safe and effective therapy of imagery utilizes the imagination and memory of meaningful experiences to promote healing. Imagery minimizes our response to stress and can reduce the symptoms of disease. When holding images that are tranquil and serene in our mind, for example, we can promote physiological and emotional relaxation. And when we visualize that health and vitality are being restored to our bodies, we enhance feelings of well-being, which in turn can reduce symptoms of illness.

We employ mental imagery when we envision a pleasant place or feeling in our minds that is so vivid it induces physiological and emotional changes. Just as the body responds to stress whether it is real or imagined, so it responds to our images, unable to discern that they are abstract! Imagery therapy provides a range of recuperative health benefits, from relaxation to pain relief, and can be an integral component of other mind-body therapies such as biofeedback (Chapter Two) and hypnosis (Chapter Eight).

Relaxation imagery seeks to induce a calm physiological

and emotional state, so that harmony in mind and body can be restored. Imagery also diminishes the stresses and tensions from body and mind, which are known to contribute to illness. It has long been known that physiological changes associated with chronic or prolonged stress have harmful effects on the body. Stress can contribute to elevated blood pressure and increase susceptibility to infections and many other diseases. During relaxation imagery, we become immersed in a calming experience. Our calm, peaceful thoughts promote a similarly calm emotional and physiological reaction. When we imagine ourselves lying on the beach on a warm, breezy day, we may begin to breathe more fully and deeply as if we were really there. Our heart rate and blood pressure will slow, and tensions will dissipate from the body. A fifteen-minute relaxation imagery practice can make us feel restored and refreshed for hours or the entire day! And because symptoms of pain and discomfort are thought to intensify while under stress, relaxation imagery can be helpful in minimizing these symptoms.

Visualization, a form of imagery, can be a strong ally in managing symptoms of chronic illnesses. Studies suggest that imagery may be used to treat a wide variety of conditions, including chronic pain, allergies, high blood pressure, irregular heartbeats, autoimmune diseases like diabetes, cold and flu, plus stress-related gastrointestinal, reproductive, and urinary complaints. It may also help to speed healing after an injury. Visualization is employed when, for example, a person with asthma paints a vivid picture in his or her mind of each bronchiole in the respiratory system opening up slowly and completely. Gradually, breathing may slow and become deeper, and symptoms may lessen. When visualization is used by cancer patients, a heightened sense of control can result, which can renew one's verve and thus increase the quality of self-care. This in turn can improve symptoms. For example, someone with cancer may visualize cancer cells waving the white flag and being swept from the body by triumphant immune-system cells. While studies don't support the claim that such a technique will strengthen the immune system, visualization can reduce anxiety and symptoms of pain, as well as increase relaxation. It also can empower the person to have a feeling of control over his or her life.

Imagery therapy is possible because the brain does not distinguish between a real or an imagined experience. Thus, the more fully you imagine an experience, the more convincing it is to the brain and the greater the physiological response. So during a day at the beach, if you can *feel* the sun blazing on your shoulders, *smell* the salty spray, and *savor* the fried clams, as far as your brain is concerned, you won't have to leave home! Also, when imagery is adapted to our particular likes and dislikes, it is more effective. For example, if the speaker on a relaxation tape asks you to envision a still, snow-covered day in a cabin at the Pocono mountains and you have arthritis that is sensitive to dampness and cold, you will certainly have difficulty relaxing! On the other hand, if you are an avid skier and live for winter adventures in the mountains, your response will differ dramatically.

Imagery may be used alone or with adjunctive therapies. When used with hypnosis, imagery can achieve a highly focused state of mind. When incorporated in a biofeedback program, imagery will relax the mind and help to alter the body's physiology. Imagery is also very effective when complementing other natural therapies like aerobic exercise, meditation, and hatha-yoga.

The description of a relaxation imagery exercise that follows is designed to help one become calm and minimize tension that may be contributing to pain. Either commit the words to memory, or record them on a cassette tape and play it during the session, or ask a friend to read the description to you. Be sure to pause between words and sentences. Eventually you will not need the tape and will be able to relax spontaneously using this or your own images.

If you have difficulty relaxing in the practice described, or you want to learn additional techniques, you may want to consult a relaxation therapist, usually a psychologist, social worker, or psychiatrist. A professional can develop an effective imagery program that is geared toward your personal preferences. However, many possibilities exist for adapting this exercise to your own personality. You might add sounds and envision images of the outdoors, of birds, or whatever else is soothing to you. If you notice that you are particularly tense in certain parts of your body, you may want to spend more time when you reach those areas in the exercise. Before beginning the exercise, practice *breathing for relaxation* (as described on pages 90–93) for several minutes. Then lie on the floor in the *corpse* pose of *hatha-yoga* (see pages 93–97). Now begin the exercise as follows:

Relaxation Imagery Technique

Choose a word like "OOH" or "UMM," and repeat it again and again, several times quietly in your mind. Let your distracting thoughts come and go without becoming involved with them. When you are in touch with the flow of the breath—that is, you can feel a movement associated with it somewhere in your body, such as in your chest or your nostrils—slow down the chanting, but quicken your pace if your thoughts begin to interfere, and slow down again only after a rhythm is reestablished. Now direct your attention to the toes of your left foot, feeling any sensations in this area.

Relax your body stage by stage, beginning from the toes. Feel a tingling in the tips of your toes and roots of your toenails. Let waves of relaxation wash into your body with every breath you take and spread to all of the parts. The waves wash into your left toe, alleviating the knots of tension. Relax your left toe . . . the sole of your left foot . . . your left ankle . . . lower leg . . . knee . . . thigh . . . hip. Relax the toes of your right foot . . . the bottom of the right foot . . . upper foot . . . ankle . . . lower leg . . . knee . . . thigh . . . hip . . . your buttocks. Let the wave wash into both legs from the toes to the hips . . . inhale deeply and chant "OOH" or your chosen word in your mind. Feel the vibrations of sound travel from your chest to your toes. Be aware of your breath rising and falling in the abdomen and chest. Feel the oxygen filling your lungs and spreading energy into all of the areas of your body each time you inhale. Let your feeling of relaxation increase with each breath. Relax your whole pelvis . . . the genitals . . . buttocks . . . rectum . . . the lower back . . . abdomen . . . the upper back . . . rib cage . . . chest . . . the shoulder blades . . . shoulders. Let the waves of relaxation wash into every part of your body, taking away the knots of tension.

Feel your right arm loosen up as the wave washes into the upper arm . . . down to your elbow . . . to the forearm . . . wrist . . . back of the hand . . . palm . . . thumb . . . fingers. Feel a tingling in the tips of your fingers, and the roots of your fingernails. Let all of the tension go from your right arms with the wave of relaxation.

Now it moves into your left arm, loosening the upper arm . . . the elbow . . . forearm . . . wrist . . . back of the hand . . . palm . . . thumb . . . fingers. Let your left fingers tingle. Let your body up to your neck float on a wave of relaxation. Now the wave moves into your neck and throat, washing all of the tension away. Now it is

slowly and gently reaching your jaw . . . chin . . . lips
. . . teeth . . . gums . . . roof of the mouth . . .
tongue . . . back of the throat . . . cheeks . . . nose.

Feel your breath move in and out of the nostrils as the
wave washes away your tension. Now it is moving to your
ears. Listen to the sound of your breath as your tension
melts away. Now it reaches your eyes . . . eyelids . . .
around the eyes . . . eyebrows . . . forehead . . . temples . . . scalp . . . and the entire skull. Inhale deeply,
and hum "UMM" or your chosen word, feeling the vibra-
tion in your throat spread through your head. Inhale, and
feel the waves of relaxation go from the tip of your toes to
the top of the skull. Now envision a sea of tranquility.
Descend further and further into the waves of relaxation.

MASSAGE

An ancient therapy embraced by Hippocrates, massage
is the door to a relaxed emotional state, but also promotes
a keen awareness of the senses found in our body. An
invigorating massage can restore the balance of energy in
the body and mind and transform a laborious day to an
uplifting evening. A relaxing massage can soothe emotional
and physiological stress and aching muscles and restore
harmony between us and the world. Specific techniques
may be used for temporarily relieving a variety of conditions, from gynecological problems to arthritis.

Massage has a host of physiological benefits. Massage
can increase the circulation without putting a strain on the
heart; it improves drainage of the lymphatic system, which
ferries toxins from the body. It can also release lactic acid
from the muscles, which causes fatigue, a process that
could take days without massage. Also, a relaxing massage
can decrease our heart rate and lower blood pressure. Jap-

anese massage, called *shiatsu*, restores the balance of energy in the body and, in the process, releases the body's natural painkilling endorphins and enkephalins.

While removing physical interferences, a massage therapist can produce another benefit by releasing blocked emotions and stress that can become manifested in the muscles. We develop certain stances to indicate our emotions—a pout to indicate brooding, for example—of which we are often unaware. A massage or body therapist can release the emotion when she or he frees the body from its physical manifestation. Other manifestations of stress can occur when our muscles become tense and throw our skeletal structure—especially the spine—into misalignment. Massage is an effective way to release muscle spasms causing misalignment and, often, pain.

Massage can be emotionally nurturing, affirming our self-esteem. The most effective form of massage is much more than the manipulation of the body's tissues; it is a connection between giver and receiver, and offers restoration to the whole person. When healing energy is exchanged, the benefits can be just as great for the giver as for the receiver. Often a meditative state of serenity is experienced by both giver and receiver during massage. A nurturing massage can increase body acceptance, a vital healing tool for those who have recently undergone surgical operations like mastectomies and for those with body-image-related difficulties like eating disorders.

Because massage heightens body awareness, it can promote better posture, improved circulation, and more efficient musculoskeletal functioning. Furthermore, increased body awareness can provide an avenue for averting physical manifestations of emotional stress, often before your mind is aware that the stress has occurred!

Massage is a popular therapy for everyone from athlete to armchair enthusiast, and many different forms have been developed to suit everyone's tastes. Swedish massage, popular at spas and sports centers, follows a set routine and is good for a general tone-up. Shiatsu massage is a Japanese therapy based on energy meridians similar to those in Chinese medicine and aims to stimulate pressure points to encourage the flow of energy (*chi*) through the body.

There are many types of strokes used in massage to achieve desired effects. In general, short, slow, and gentle strokes aid lymphatic drainage beneath the skin, while deeper strokes are used to release tension in muscles. Percussion is used to stimulate the body, while light, feathery strokes are very effective in achieving relaxation.

Clothing is worn for shiatsu massage, and oil is not used. During other forms of massage, oil is applied to the bare skin. In general, you should keep your hands in contact with the body as much as possible when giving a massage. Part of the therapeutic effect of massage lies in its nurturing human contact, and an abrupt or rote pounding of the tissues may convey quite the opposite message. A gentle, continuous flow of contact between giver and receiver is the best way to restore harmony to body and mind. Don't be afraid to cause slight discomfort during certain portions of massage. A certain degree of pain is beneficial for releasing tension from aching or stiff muscles. If pain is severe or persistent, however, another underlying and serious condition may be present. In this case, consult a physician or a chiropractor immediately.

Precautions: Do not massage areas of open wounds or bruises or varicose veins, swelling, or inflammation due to injury. A massage should not be given to someone who has a fever.

Massage can be used in conjunction with any alternative therapy, and is often combined with acupressure, aromatherapy, and chiropractic. For additional applications using essential oils, see aromatherapy.

Massage Warmup

To begin, apply oil to the side of the body that you're working on. Apply long, gliding strokes to familiarize yourself with the body and to stimulate the energy between you and the recipient. Use whatever oils seem to suit the skin. Cold-pressed vegetable oils that contain B and E vitamins are easily absorbed. Grapeseed, safflower, and sweet-almond oils are lighter than wheat-germ, olive, and avocado oils. The latter group, when mixed with a lighter oil, are beneficial for dry skin. For skin that is oily, inflamed, or has acne, use jojoba oil, which is not actually an oil but a wax.

Begin with the face, stroking the forehead, then the cheeks, with the thumbs, pushing out from the center to each side of the face. At the neck, using one thumb, work down one side at a time, applying pressure at equal intervals. To massage the shoulders, use a kneading motion of the fingers to apply pressure to them. You will relieve knots of tension and feel the tissue become softer and more pliable. To massage the arms, first apply long, gliding strokes, then squeeze gently with the fingers. When you reach the hands, pull on each finger gently. On the back of the palms, use your palm to rub in a clockwise motion. Next is the chest. Apply long, gliding strokes, then use the heels of the palm to rub small circles.

To massage the legs, begin with the feet and work up to the thighs, squeezing gently with the fingers. Apply pressure with the thumb to the inside back of the ankle and to the back of the thigh. Both improve circulation. The ankle pressure should help to relieve fluid retention. Rub the sole of the foot from heel to toe with a gliding motion to improve circulation. Gently pull on each toe. When you finish, lightly brush your fingers over this side of the body for a relaxing effect.

Now apply oil to the other side of the body, and repeat the same techniques for the neck and arms. To massage the back, first apply long, gliding strokes. Then begin at the upper part of the spine, and, using both thumbs side by side, apply pressure about a half-inch away from the spine, working down one side of it. Use a fast movement for a stimulating effect and a slow movement for a relaxing effect. Finish at the coccyx (the end of the spine), then begin again, working down the other side of the spine. Try to apply pressure at the same intervals on both sides. Now move to the buttocks, and gently knead them with your fingers. Massage the legs just as on the other side. When you finish, lightly brush your fingers over the whole side of the body for a relaxing effect.

MEDITATION

Once thought of as the exclusive practice of Zen monks and Hindu yogis, meditation was popularized in America during the 1960s when studies revealed its powerful physiological and emotional effects. A valuable therapy for those with hectic lives, meditation promotes deep physiological relaxation and has many other applications, from managing stress to reducing pain.

Meditation is a non-activity, a state of mindful awareness in which our thoughts and actions play no role. When machines monitor people in the quiet, meditative state, profound differences are recorded from those who sit quietly or sleep. Heart and breathing rates are vastly slowed, oxygen consumption drops, and blood hormonal levels are influenced. In addition, psychological changes can often be noted. Anxiety, hostility, and aggression are reduced, self-esteem improved, energy elevated, and physical stamina increased.

Because of its value in promoting relaxation, meditation is the perfect antidote for the complicated, stressful lifestyle. Stress has been recognized as an increased risk for many diseases, as well as an important influence on our experience of symptoms and illness. Calm, peaceful thoughts, for example, tend to lead to a similar emotional reaction and comparable physiological reactions, while angry or anxious thoughts tend to incite us emotionally, leading to a greater physiological response. The quiet state of meditation counteracts tension by promoting tranquility of the mind, which relaxes the body. During gynecological discomforts, from menstruation to menopause, meditation can provide great relief from emotional symptoms of irritability, anxiety, and tension. With practice, it can even be used to reduce the sensation of pain and discomfort. In addition, study results have shown that stress-reduction strategies, when practiced regularly, can raise the threshold of provocation leading to a stress response.

Meditation has been used as the primary therapy in pain management of some cases. People with chronic and painful illnesses learn to use the meditative state to learn to live better with pain. The here-and-now philosophy of meditation helps a person recognize and let go of anxious thoughts that can heighten sensations of pain, thus transforming the sensation of pain into a bearable and even uneventful experience.

There are many types of meditation, and each provides roughly the same results. Some forms of meditation like that used in Zen Buddhism and Hinduism incorporate religious beliefs. However, it is not necessary to observe such faiths to practice these meditative styles. Another style is called Transcendental Meditation. Group practice of Zen meditation is sometimes offered free of charge at a local community center and typically involves some religious observance. The group experience can heighten the meditative experience for participants. Check at your local university or college for listings. Weekend and week-long retreats are available for all forms of meditation.

Below is a practice mediation you can do for 15 minutes every day. Wear loose clothing and sit in quiet surroundings. Practice *breathing for relaxation* (as described on pages 90–93) before you begin, and try to incorporate the breathing technique throughout the exercise. Don't worry about following the practice closely—you can adapt it to suit your own tastes. Once you learn the ropes, you may want to practice meditation twice each day. Practice during short breaks at the office (if you can find a quiet place), or as a transition between the office and a relaxed evening. Meditation can be combined with other mind-body therapies like biofeedback (Chapter Two), imagery, hypnosis (Chapter Eight), psychotherapy (Chapter Two), and virtually any other natural therapy.

Practice Meditation

You can perform the following meditation to experience "mindfulness." Read it first, and then try to meditate without referring to the text. It's more important to relax than it is to follow these instructions closely. You can perform the following meditation while sitting on the floor with legs crossed and feet tucked in as close to your body as possible. Keep your back straight and rest your hands on your knees. You can also sit in a chair or kneel on the floor sitting back on your calves. The practice will take approximately fifteen minutes, but you can expand or shorten it to suit your needs. Every person's experience of meditation can vary, so don't be concerned if you do not undergo the experience described here.

Choose a word, and chant it to yourself. You can use a religious word like "God" or a more secular word like "one." Do not say the word out loud, but listen to its sound in your mind. Listen to the sound over and over again in your mind as you let your thoughts come and let them go. When you are in touch with the rhythm of the sound and you can feel its resonance somewhere in your body, such as in your toes or fingers, slow down the chanting, but quicken your pace if your thoughts begin to interfere, and slow down again only after a rhythm is reestablished. Now listen to the chanting gradually grow louder in your body. First its sound may be somewhat hushed and barely felt in the arms, the trunk, and the legs. It may grow more audible and swell into other parts of the body—up to the forehead and down to the ankles. With each breathing sequence, the sound may ring in your body two or three times. It may begin to boom, gush into your toes and fingers and every crevice of your body. Then it may taper somewhat suddenly and disappear from your body. In the silence, notice your thoughts come and go, without becoming distracted by them. If you do become distracted, begin chanting again. Conclude by wishing prosperity and health to all of humanity.

NUTRITIONAL THERAPY

As the evidence of food's power to make or break illness grows, more and more people are turning to the kitchen cupboard instead of the medicine cabinet for the tools of better health. Increasingly evident is food's power to hinder the onset of certain illnesses like cancer, heart disease, and osteoporosis and to minimize the symptoms of various gynecological discomforts, among other conditions. With such promising evidence, food may very well be the therapy of the twenty-first century.

While its benefits are evident, nutritional therapy can be a problem for those of us who have difficulty in breaking the bad habits learned over the years—habits that, unfortunately, don't break themselves. As teenagers, we learned to eat "empty calories," foods containing few of the precious vitamins and minerals so essential to disease prevention. As adults, we don't find the time to steam vegetables and trim fat from our meat because we're just plain too busy.

Such are the thought processes behind poor eating habits for most of us. However, if we thought of healthy food as a magic charm that would grant us three wishes—health, happiness, and longevity, perhaps?—we would well consider postponing a shopping excursion to stop by the grocery store for the much-exalted fruits and vegetables, wouldn't we? All fantasies aside, the truth is that food *is* that magic charm. Fibrous fresh fruits and vegetables have been linked with lower incidence of certain cancers. Potassium-rich foods reduce risks for heart disease and strokes. Cystitis can be healed with cranberries and vaginitis with yogurt. The kitchen cupboard has many other applications as well, from menstrual relief to stress reduction.

Also, remember that once you invest the time in developing new eating habits, maintenance time will be minimal. Once developed, eating habits will become second nature, and if you regularly eat nutritious food, you likely won't have much desire to eat other things. You'll be reducing your risk for developing numerous diseases, and you'll feel better than ever!

The following are good food sources for the nutrients required for essential body processes. Also listed is the daily U.S. recommended dietary allowance of each nutrient for adult women.

Water-Soluble Vitamins

- *Vitamin C (ascorbic acid):* citrus fruits, strawberries, cantaloupe, potatoes, green and red peppers, broccoli, cauliflower, snow peas, cabbage, sweet potatoes, watermelon, plantains, and tomatoes. U.S. RDA—60 milligrams.

- *Bioflavonoids:* grapes, rose hips, prunes, oranges, lemon juice, cherries, black currants, plums, parsley, cabbage, apricots, peppers, papaya, cantaloupe, tomatoes, broccoli, and blackberries. U.S. RDA—not set.

B-Complex Vitamins

- B_1 *(thiamine):* fortified grains and cereals, seafood, and pork. U.S. RDA—1 milligram.

- B_2 *(riboflavin):* low-fat dairy products, fortified cereals and grains, organ meats, beef, lamb, dark meat of poultry, and dark green, leafy vegetables. U.S. RDA— 1.2 to 1.3 milligrams.

- B_3 *(niacin):* poultry and seafood, seeds, nuts, peanuts, potatoes, and fortified whole-grain breads and cereals. U.S. RDA—13 to 15 milligrams.

- B_5 *(pantothenic acid):* found in almost all plant and animal foods; also manufactured in the intestine. U.S. RDA—5 to 10 milligrams.

- *PABA (para-aminobenzoic acid):* molasses, brewer's yeast, eggs, whole grains, and wheat germ. U.S. RDA —not set.

- *B_6 (pyridoxine):* grains and cereals—especially brown rice—spinach, sweet potatoes, bananas, pears, white potatoes, prunes, watermelon, meats, fish, and poultry. U.S. RDA—1.6 milligrams.

- *B_{12} (cobalamin):* all animal products, including meats, eggs, poultry, seafood, and low-fat dairy products. U.S. RDA—2 milligrams.

- *Biotin:* manufactured in the intestine; also found in meats, poultry, fish, eggs, nuts, seeds, legumes, oranges, tomatoes, raspberries, and grapefruit. U.S. RDA—150 to 300 micrograms (a microgram is one millionth of a gram).

- *Folic acid:* poultry, liver, dark-green leafy vegetables, legumes, fortified whole-grain cereals and breads, and orange and grapefruit juice. U.S. RDA—180 milligrams.

Fat-Soluble Vitamins

- *Vitamin A:* yellow vegetables and fruits, including carrots, pumpkin, mangoes, sweet potatoes, yellow squash, and corn; also spinach, broccoli, beet greens, eggs, whole-milk products, and fish oils. (Beta-carotene, the precursor to vitamin A, is found in plant sources and is not toxic. Vitamin A, however, is toxic in very high amounts.) U.S. RDA—800 RE (one RE = 1 microgram of retinol or 6 micrograms of beta-carotene).

- *Vitamin D:* egg yolks, fish and cod-liver oil, and fortified milk and butter. U.S. RDA—5 milligrams.

- *Vitamin E:* poultry, seafood, green leafy vegetables, nuts, seeds, eggs, wheat germ, wheat-germ oil, and fortified cereals. U.S. RDA—8 milligrams.

- *Vitamin K:* manufactured in the intestine; also found in yogurt, soy products, kale, spinach, cauliflower, broccoli, and cabbage. U.S. RDA—not set.

Macro Minerals

- *Calcium:* dairy products, oysters, certain types of tofu, dark-green leafy vegetables like broccoli and brussels sprouts, collard greens, sea vegetables like kelp, pumpkin and sesame seeds, corn tortillas, oatmeal, salmon, herring, almonds, peanuts with skins left on them, hazelnuts, calcium-fortified soy milk, and soy powder for making a milk substitute. U.S. RDA—800 milligrams.

- *Magnesium:* green leafy vegetables, beans, nuts, seeds, avocados, turnips, fortified whole-grain cereals and breads, oysters, scallops, carob, honey, and blackstrap molasses. U.S. RDA—280 milligrams.

- *Phosphorus:* dairy products, egg yolks, meat, poultry, fish, whole grains, legumes, celery, cabbage, carrots, pumpkin, cucumber, and chard. U.S. RDA—800 milligrams.

Trace Minerals

- *Iron:* legumes, dried apricots, raisins, peaches, cherries, figs, dates, prunes, fortified breads and cereals, blackstrap molasses, pumpkin seeds, torula yeast, rice bran, red meat and liver, egg yolks, shellfish and fish, and acidic foods cooked in cast-iron pots. U.S. RDA— 15 milligrams.

- *Zinc:* oysters, yogurt, fortified cereals, wheat germ, peas, soybeans, mushrooms, most nuts and seeds— especially pumpkin seeds—beef, and liver. U.S. RDA —12 milligrams.

- *Iodine:* sea vegetables such as kelp, fresh seafood, garlic, dried mushrooms, green leafy vegetables, celery, tomatoes, carrots, radishes, and onions. U.S. RDA— 150 milligrams.

- *Copper:* lobster, organ meats, nuts, dried peas, beans, prunes, and barley. U.S. RDA—not set.

- *Chromium:* nuts, black pepper, whole grains except rye and corn, fresh fruit juices, dairy products, root vegetables, leafy vegetables, legumes, and mushrooms. U.S. RDA—not set.

- *Selenium:* whole grains, mushrooms, asparagus, broccoli, onions, tomatoes, and eggs. U.S. RDA—not set.

- *Manganese:* tea, coffee, bran, dried peas and beans, and nuts. U.S. RDA—not set.

- *Potassium:* green leafy vegetables, bananas, cantaloupes, avocados, dates, prunes, dried apricots, raisins, oranges, potatoes, whole grains, beans, legumes, nuts, and seeds.

- *Sodium:* table salt and processed foods.

Vegetarian Protein Sources

- *Partial proteins:* corn, legumes (beans, chick peas, lentils, peas, peanuts, soybeans), tofu, whole grains of all kinds, nuts and seeds (pumpkin, sesame, and sunflower) yogurt, milk, and cheese.

- *Complete proteins:* millet, whole grains with legumes (e.g., rice with beans, rice with lentils), nuts or seeds with legumes (e.g., pea soup with pumpkin-seed topping), nuts or seeds with whole grains (e.g., bread with sunflower or sesame seeds), milk products with legumes (e.g., peanut-butter sandwich and milk), milk products with whole grains (e.g., cheese sandwich), and milk products with nuts or seeds (e.g., cheese ball rolled in sesame seeds). U.S. RDA for protein—46 grams.

Water-Soluble Fiber

Water-soluble fiber is found in fresh fruits and vegetables, oat bran, and legumes.

Insoluble Fiber

Insoluble fiber is found in bran from whole grains besides oat.

Saturated and Unsaturated Fats

- *Saturated fats:* These raise blood cholesterol levels. They include butter and beef fat, and are found in all dairy products like cheese, yogurt, and milk. Palm, palm kernel, and coconut oils, also saturated, are used in many pastries and sweets because they're inexpensive.

- *Polyunsaturated fats:* These lower blood cholesterol. They include cottonseed, corn, safflower, soybean, sunflower oils, fish-lipid oils, wheat-germ oil, black-currant oil, and gamma-linolenic acid.

- *Monounsaturated fats:* These also lower blood cholesterol. They include canola, peanut, olive, and sesame-seed oils.

Gamma-Linolenic Acid

Gamma-linolenic acid (GLA) is found in nuts, seeds, avocadoes, fresh fish, and cold-pressed olive and sunflower oils. It can also be extracted from seeds of some plants, like the evening primrose and black currants (see "Nutritional Therapy," Chapter Four).

Linoleic Acid

Linoleic acid is found in Brazil nuts, pumpkin and squash seeds, peanut butter, sunflower seeds, sesame oil, corn oil, safflower oil, cottonseed oil, almonds, Spanish peanuts, black walnuts, and English walnuts.

CHAPTER FOUR

Menstrual Problems

Women who suffer from pain and discomfort related to menstruation, an estimated 75 million in the United States, may have the most to gain from natural therapies. While physicians of the past dismissed premenstrual symptoms of pain, nausea, and other discomforts as a psychological illness with no organic basis, medical opinion on the subject has since evolved. In recent years, the allopathic community has acknowledged that premenstrual syndrome (PMS) and menstrual pain are complex biochemical processes that can be influenced by a range of lifestyle factors including diet, exercise, emotional health, social support, and stress. Still, many women seeking treatment from allopathic physicians walk from the doctor's office feeling frustrated. Allopathic treatment for PMS, except with strong prescription drugs, simply doesn't exist.

Menstrual symptoms are one of many challenges that natural therapies can rise to meet, since lifestyle and the whole person are so integral to treatment. Proper holistic care can soothe and revitalize the person, maximize health, and prevent recurrence of menstrual pain. In this chapter you will learn about healing herbs that relieve these discomforts with soothing natural chemicals that mimic a woman's own hormones, thereby providing a natural "replacement" therapy; and about therapies like aerobic exercise and yoga that produce relief by stimulating natural physiological changes that comfort both mind and body. Aerobic exercise causes the body to release natural pain-killing hormones that are deficient during menstruation. And yoga can provide mental release from pain. Ancient healing techniques such as acupressure and acupuncture release and redirect vital energy (*chi*) that restores and bolsters health, and, in the process, activates natural pain-killing chemicals.

You already have an idea of how most of these therapies work, so our discussion will turn to specific applications for relieving menstrual problems. But first let us look more closely at the menstrual cycle that takes place each month during a woman's fertile years.

At menarche, a woman has some 75,000 follicles that will mature into eggs. Each month in the years between menarche and menopause the body prepares to release one or more of those eggs for possible fertilization. Hormones are released by the ovaries that cause changes in the uterus, preparing it to support a fetus. The uterine lining, called the endometrium, thickens from the growth of blood vessels and other nutrients. Finally, the ovaries release an egg into the fallopian tubes for possible impregnation by a sperm. If the egg is not fertilized, the body's response is menstruation, during which the uterine lining is shed. This cycle typically lasts twenty-eight days, but can be as short as twenty or as long as thirty-six days. Menstruation may last from four to six days, but can span from two to eight days. Painful symptoms can be experienced from two to three days to several weeks.

Many practitioners believe that hormonal fluctuations during menstruation are the culprits causing pain and discomfort. During the menstrual cycle, the ovaries secrete levels of the hormone estrogen, then the hormone progesterone, which prepare the uterus for pregnancy. Prior to menstruation, hormones drop sharply, causing the uterus to shed its lining. Other hormonal changes occur prior to menstruation, including a dip in the body's painkilling endorphins and enkephalins.

Symptoms experienced during this cycle can range from the neurological to the psychological, varying from woman to woman, by age, and from month to month. Generally speaking, symptoms will lessen in severity once women reach their thirties and after childbirth, because pregnancy usually increases the network of blood vessels to the uterus. Some women experience only mild discomfort, while others are debilitated during menstruation. Milder symptoms include swelling or tenderness of breasts, fluid retention, slight enlargement in the abdominal area and some twinges of pain. But many women experience more severe symptoms of tension, irritability, anxiety, hostility, crying spells, lethargy, depression, insomnia, tension headaches and neck aches, migraines, dizziness, fainting, constipation, abdominal bloating, abdominal cramping, and "sweet tooth" cravings.

While no one knows exactly what the biochemical basis is for menstrual-cycle symptoms, and indeed these physiological processes affect each woman differently, there are many commonly held theories. These include hormonal changes, salt or water retention, a low-nutrient diet, deficiencies of magnesium or vitamin B_6, psychosocial factors, including depression, and lack of aerobic exercise. In addition, factors like strenuous exercise, increased sexual activity, the use of an IUD (intrauterine device) or birth control pills may cause irregular menstrual periods. The start of menopause may also lead to abnormal menstrual flow and erratic periods (see Chapter Seven).

It's important to recognize that strong menstrual cramps after years without them, or heavy bleeding, can be warning signs of other serious conditions. If periods suddenly become painful after years without discomfort, it could be a sign of endometriosis. When pain worsens toward the end of your period, you may have fibroids (see Chapter Five). Prolonged, early, or heavy periods, especially with mild fever and odorous vaginal discharge, could be a sign of pelvic infection. If any of these symptoms develop, see your physician immediately because they could require antibiotics or other serious medical treatment. (For more information, see Chapter Five.)

In general, it is likely that a combination of factors produces menstrual symptoms in each woman and consequently that several avenues of therapy should be pursued for relief. You will experience varying success rates with different therapies, so experimenting with different treatments will enhance your overall comfort. This will also help you to learn more about the causes of your condition.

ACUPRESSURE/ACUPUNCTURE

The time-tested energy therapies of acupressure and acupuncture often provide the key to solving many women's gynecological problems. While the emphasis is on prevention, illness can arise when energy imbalance arises in any of the fourteen meridians. Most menstrual problems, as well as most other female gynecological problems have been linked with three specific meridians—of the spleen, kidney, and liver—and treatment is usually to one or all of these pathways and connected energy systems. Causes of these imbalances may include such lifestyle practices as repeated exposure to cold climates (unheated living quarters, running in the winter during menses), consumption of excessive amounts of cold foods (including ice creams, frozen desserts, raw salads, fruit juices), emotional stress, overwork, and overall feebleness of vital energy (*chi*) or the blood. Premenstrual problems can result from sluggishness or stagnation of energy caused by the life-style practices mentioned above as well as the overconsumption of caffeine, alcohol, and sugar, repressed emotions, and lack of exercise.

Acupressure treatment involves a variety of point-stimulation techniques that redirect the flow of energy in the body, and, in the process, prompt secretion of the body's most potent painkillers, endorphins and enkephalins. Points are often chosen *local* to the discomfort as well as *distal* to it. Distal points are usually located on the arms below the elbow and on the legs below the knees. The distal points are often (but not always) on the same meridian where the pain or discomfort occurs. Holding both points simultaneously creates an energy circuit that encourages the energy to normalize. Since this may be difficult to accomplish during self-treatment, it is best to seek treatment from a licensed acupuncturist or trained acupressure therapist. Acupuncture has been found to be effective in treating a wide variety of menstrual problems, including amenorrhea (lack of periods), irregular periods, heavy periods, cramping, clotting, and premenstrual symptoms. Usually, gynecological problems are treated over the course of three menstrual cycles. These treatments should be adequate to provide relief for months from menstrual pain and discomfort. For more information, see "Acupuncture," Chapter Three.

Described below are various acupressure remedies for common menstrual complaints. Unless otherwise noted, you should press each acupressure point with firm but gentle pressure for two to three minutes, or until you feel relief. You will have to train yourself to place your attention in your fingertips! For further instructions on how to apply acupressure, see "Acupressure," Chapter Three.

While acupressure is a gentle, safe treatment when used correctly, some precautions should be taken. You should never use acupressure as a *primary* treatment to relieve excessive bleeding, vaginal discharges, or undiagnosed pain, each of which can be an indication of serious illness requiring prompt medical care.

For Irritability

- *Liver 3:* This point is located on the top of the foot in the depression beyond the juncture of the metatarsal bones of the big toe and the second toe.
- *Large intestine 4:* You'll feel this acupressure point in the upper part of the web between the thumb and forefinger on the back of the hand.

For Breast Tenderness

- *Stomach 34:* Find this point two finger-widths above the tip of kneecap on its outside edge.
- *Liver 3:* This point is located on the top of the foot in the depression beyond the juncture of the metatarsal bones of the big toe and the second toe.
- *Conception vessel 17:* You'll find this point at the center of the breastbone at the level of the fourth rib.
- *Pericardium 6:* You can locate this point about three finger-widths from upper crease of the wrist on the inner forearm between the two tendons.
- *Stomach 18:* You'll feel this point in the space between the fifth and sixth rib directly below the nipple.

For Fluid Retention

- *Conception vessel 9:* This point is located about one thumb-width directly above the bellybutton.
- *Kidney 3:* Locate this point on the inside of the ankle between the Achilles tendon and the ankle bone.

For Menstrual Pain and Discomfort

- *Bladder 32:* You'll feel this point in the second sacral foramen of the lower spine on either side.
- *Liver 3:* This point is located on the top of the foot in the depression beyond the juncture of the metatarsal bones of the big toe and the second toe.
- *Spleen 8:* Locate this point about three inches or four finger-widths below the head of the tibia, on the inside of the calf. Press against the bone. (It may be helpful to view the diagram at the back of the book.)
- *Stomach 36:* This point is located on the calf, four finger-widths below the bottom of the kneecap, one finger-width on the outside of the shinbone. The point is on a muscle, so you'll know you're in the right place if you can feel it move when you flex your foot.
- *Conception vessel 4:* Feel for this point about four finger-widths directly below the bellybutton, or about two thumb-widths above the pubic bone.
- *Conception vessel 6:* Find this point two finger-widths below the bellybutton.
- *Spleen 6:* You can find this point by placing four fingers above the ankle on the inside of the leg, right behind the shinbone. Either calming or strengthening will work here to relieve cramps.

Heavy Menstruation

- *Kidney 3:* Locate this point on the inside of the ankle between the Achilles tendon and the anklebone.

- *Spleen 1:* This point is situated where the nail of the big toe meets the skin, at the bottom inside corner (e.g., the right side of your right foot). Besides pressing this point, a very effective way to stop heavy bleeding is to hold an incense stick near the point until it is hot. Move the incense stick away briefly, then repeat again to reheat the point. Note: this point is generally effective only during menstruation.

- *Conception vessel 4:* Feel for this point about four finger-widths directly below the bellybutton, or two finger-widths above the pubic bone.

- *Spleen 6:* You can find this point by placing four fingers above the ankle on the inside of the leg, right behind the shinbone. Either calming or strengthening will work here to relieve cramps.

- *Conception vessel 6:* Find this point two finger-widths below the bellybutton.

- *Stomach 36:* This point is located on the calf, four finger-widths below the bottom of the kneecap, one finger-width on the outside of the shinbone. The point is on a muscle, so you'll know you're in the right place if you can feel it move when you flex your foot.

For Nausea and Sweet-Tooth Cravings

- *Spleen 6:* You can find this point by placing four fingers above the ankle on the inside of the leg, right behind the shinbone. Either calming or strengthening will work here to relieve cramps.

- *Stomach 36:* This point is located on the calf, four finger-widths below the bottom of the kneecap, one finger-width on the outside of the shinbone. The point is on a muscle, so you'll know you're in the right place if you can feel it move when you flex your foot.

- *Pericardium 6:* You can locate this point about three finger-widths from upper crease of the wrist on the inner forearm between the two tendons.

For Insomnia or Depression

- *Liver 3:* This point is located on the top of the foot in the depression beyond the juncture of the metatarsal bones of the big toe and the second toe.

- *Anmian:* Below the skull on the posterior edge of the mastoid, midway between *gall bladder 20* (see Chapter Seven) and the depression behind the earlobe.

- *Spleen 6:* Locate this point about four finger-widths up from the inside anklebone right behind the shinbone.

- *Pericardium 6:* You can locate this point about three finger-widths from upper crease of the wrist on the inner forearm.

- *Heart 7:* With the palm up, this point is located on the wrist crease on the smallest-finger side. Press under the tendons. This point is especially helpful in relieving emotional symptoms of anxiety and irritability.

- *Yintang:* You'll find this point between the eyes, right above the nose.

AEROBIC EXERCISE

Aerobic exercise can relieve some of the most common and most bothersome menstrual complaints like fluid retention, cramps, anxiety, irritability, and food cravings. While there are many theories about what promotes menstrual complaints, one particularly credible premise is that levels of the body's own painkilling endorphins and enkephalins dramatically drop prior to menstruation. The lack of the "feel-good" hormones brings on a range of emotional upset, from feelings of irritability to anxiety, and can exacerbate pain. A safe and easy remedy, aerobic exercise causes the body to release endorphins and enkephalins, thereby relieving pain and irritability. Swelling and fluid retention are also diminished during exercise, because the body sheds fluid to cool itself during increased activity. Finally, exercise diminishes appetite, at least temporarily, and provides a break from the "hungry horrors," intense cravings for sweets and carbohydrates. During exercise, and for at least one or two hours after, you usually will not feel hungry. However, your appetite will return and possibly may be greater than before your workout. When combined with hatha-yoga, meditation, or any other mind-body therapy, exercise may be a helpful tool in gaining control over the desire to indulge in food "binges."

If you've never exercised before, or if it has been at least several months since you've worked out, it's best to start with a walking program, gradually increasing your pace. To learn how to establish a walking or running regimen, see "Aerobic Exercise," Chapter Three.

For another natural exercise remedy during menstruation, see "Hatha-Yoga."

AROMATHERAPY

The remarkable physiological and emotional effects that are evoked by the powerful healing properties of essential oils can be quite useful for relieving menstrual problems. Menstruation is a difficult time emotionally and physically, and the essential oils found in plants can provide just the soothing relief necessary to rebalance mind and body.

Listed below are suggested remedies for common menstrual complaints. Unless otherwise noted, you should notice results right away and do not need to continue therapy after your condition is improved. Once balance and health are restored, however, you may want to incorporate into your daily routine a preventive treatment for keeping the body and spirit well. (See "Aromatherapy," Chapter Three.)

For General Premenstrual Complaints (like Fatigue, Irritability, Cramps)

Bath. Use two drops each of the following oils in a daily bath while the symptoms occur: rosemary, lavender, and chamomile, plus four drops of lemon. Submerge in a warm bath containing three drops each of pine, chamomile, and neroli oils. This bath treatment soothes and provides a maximum of relief for pain and discomfort.

Massage. This massage can have an overall restorative effect when premenstrual symptoms occur: Mix four drops of chamomile oil and three drops of neroli oil with one ounce of vegetable oil. Ask a friend to massage this into your abdomen, lower back and the back of your neck. To massage the body, first apply oil on the side you're working. Begin with the neck, and, using one thumb, work down one side at a time, applying pressure at equal intervals. To massage the lower back, begin at the lower curve of the spine, and, using both thumbs side by side, apply pressure about one thumb-width from the spine, working down one side of it to the coccyx (end of the spine). Quicker movements will stimulate, while slower movements will relax. Now work down the other side of the spine. Try to apply pressure at the same intervals on each side. Apply oil to the other side of the body. To massage the abdomen, use the palm of your hand to rub in a clockwise motion.

For Menstrual Pain

Massage. Make a massage oil from five drops of parsley oil, two drops of chamomile oil, and one drop of pine oil in an ounce of vegetable oil. Apply to the abdomen.

For Edema (Swelling)

Massage. Massage the soles of the feet with an oil consisting of three teaspoons of wheat-germ or vegetable oil and two drops each of cypress and rosemary oils. Apply oil to the skin and rub it in lightly. Use the knuckles of one hand and press firmly to rub up and down from heel to arch in one even motion.

Massage the legs with an oil consisting of a base of two ounces vegetable oil and four drops wheat-germ oil, plus three drops each of rosemary and lemon oils. Apply oil to the legs. Beginning with the feet and working up to the thighs, squeeze gently with the fingers. Apply pressure with the thumb to the inside back of the ankle and to the back of the thigh. Both improve circulation. The ankle pressure should help to relieve fluid retention.

Twice each day, rub the top of the hands, soles of the feet, the abdomen, and the solar plexus (between the ribs) with a massage oil made from the vegetable and wheat-germ mixture, plus three drops each of basil, cedarwood, cypress, and lavender oils. To massage solar plexus and tops of hands, apply oil, and use the palm of your hand to rub in a clockwise motion.

For Diarrhea

Poultice. For quick relief, make a steaming hot linseed poultice for the abdomen. Mash three to four ounces of linseeds and enough hot water to make a paste. Mix in four drops of thyme oil. While still hot, spoon the whole mixture onto the center of a piece of gauze and fold both sides of the cloth over the mixture. Apply immediately to the skin.

For Constipation

Massage. Mix together three teaspoons of wheat-germ oil and six drops of rosemary oil and massage this into the abdomen each day while symptoms occur.

For Insomnia

Bath. Lavender is a gentle narcotic that can relax us even on the most taxing days. Take a warm bath before going to bed using six drops of lavender oil.

Massage. Prepare a massage oil using one ounce of vegetable oil with two drops neroli, lavender, and melissa oils, and apply to shoulders, solar plexus, and abdomen.

For Heavy Periods or Abnormal Bleeding

Massage.   Make a massage oil of two drops each of cinnamon, juniper, pine, and geranium oils and five drops of cypress in a vegetable-oil base. Apply to lower back and abdomen.

To Regulate Cycles and Reduce Heavy Bleeding

Massage.   Make a massage oil of two drops each of chamomile, melissa, lavender, and rose or jasmine. Apply to lower back and abdomen.

To Bring on Menstrual Period and Encourage Flow

Massage.   Make a massage oil of one drop each of basil, chamomile, clary sage, juniper, lavender, marjoram, and rosemary. Apply to lower back and abdomen.

For Emotional Upset

See "Aromatherapy," Chapter Three.

BREATHING FOR RELAXATION

Reclaiming this healthful habit, which many of us have "unlearned," can reap immediate benefits. Stress and anxiety are known to have harmful effects on the body, contributing to the development of many conditions and illnesses, but menstrual sufferers may benefit most from how stress reduction influences the experience of symptoms and illness. Discomfort related to the menstrual cycle is thought to have a psychosocial component, and reducing anxiety can help to alleviate it.

While researchers are currently exploring the role that certain emotions and psychosocial factors may play in illness, it has been established that physiological changes associated with chronic or prolonged stress have harmful effects on the body. Our physiological experience of stress is called the "fight or flight" response, and changes in breathing quality—that is, rapid, shallow breathing—are one of the first and the most obvious signs that the body is launching a stress response. By interrupting the rapid-breathing response, we can slow or even avert the stress response and those harmful metabolic changes. We can also improve our experience during menstruation. Learning how to breath healthfully is the first step in managing stress. Try the belly-breathing practice described in "Breathing for Relaxation," Chapter Three.

CHIROPRACTIC

The primary-care profession of chiropractic is utilized worldwide for its natural, drug-free, surgery-free approach. Chiropractic advocates maintenance of the body's skeletal structure, primarily the spine and nervous system, to protect and restore health. Disease or discomfort can result when any number of factors cause the spinal joints, which protect nerves in the spinal cord, to be locked or out of place, upsetting the balance in the body. Misalignment can also cause reduced blood flow, pain, and discomfort, and can affect an array of other body functions, from the physiological to the emotional.

Chiropractic often provides the answer to ailments that allopathic medicine cannot treat. Illness can result when the energy interference resulting from spinal misalignment throws off the whole body by irritating nerves. It upsets the body's balance and harmony, or what is called *homeostasis*, primarily because of nerve interference. Homeostasis allows synchronicity of body functions. When interference occurs, one function in the body may take over the job of an injured body part, which can lead to overwork. For example, a weakness in the heart may cause an overstress of the lungs, which are forced to work overtime to bring in extra oxygen to make up for the weakness. This can cause a chain reaction that can continue indefinitely until the entire body system becomes unbalanced, weak, and prone to degenerative diseases.

Displacement of the lumbar spine is sometimes the culprit causing menstrual pain, when the nerves linked with the reproductive organs become irritated. Such symptoms result from changes that occur in the soft tissues surrounding the area of displacement where these nerves exit the spinal cord. When the flow of blood and lymph in nearby vessels is slowed, they become sluggish, disrupting the exchange of nutrients and waste products throughout the circulatory and lymphatic systems. The outcome is swelling, lack of oxygen, and the buildup of toxins; similarly, muscles malfunction and the nerves are often irritated. The cumulative effect of these changes is overall pain and discomfort.

Structural imbalance is often the result of childbirth, but may also be precipitated by muscle spasm, injury, bone malformation, tumor, or cysts. When muscles tense up during stress, they can throw the spine out of alignment, causing discomfort and illness. When menstrual pains are severe after years without much pain, however, it may be a warning that another condition like endometriosis, infection, or cancer has developed (see Chapter Five and Chapter Eight). You should consult a physician immediately.

If menstrual problems are the result of misalignment, the key to restoring harmony in body and mind lies in the chiropractor's highly trained hands, which provide corrective adjustments to realign bones and minimize pressure on spinal nerves. Of course, the body can correct some of its misalignments by itself even without our being aware. But when pain and tension occur with movement, you should consult a chiropractor.

During an appointment, a chiropractor, like other holistic practitioners, will discuss your health in great detail. Before diagnosing your condition, a chiropractor will observe how you walk, sit, and stand, and look for any unusual movements. She or he will also administer orthopedic and neurological tests to evaluate your coordination and reflexes. Because many bone conditions, such as hairline fractures and bone degeneration, are not visible to the eye, a chiropractor commonly uses X rays as a diagnostic aid to assess spinal health. Chiropractors also use a range of other diagnostic and treatment tools that are also employed by neurologists and physiatrists (rehabilitation specialists). An electrical muscle stimulator prevents painful spasms by emulating proper nerve impulses to the muscles. Cryogenic (cold) and heat therapies such as ultrasound and therapeutic massage complement adjustments.

Once your condition is diagnosed, your treatment may involve not only spinal manipulation, but also a recommendation for a healthier diet, stress-management techniques, or a rehabilitative exercise program. To restore spinal health, your chiropractor may employ a variety of techniques that require great precision and delicacy. Just as surgery requires extensive training and experience, so do the techniques of chiropractic. Unlike invasive surgery, however, chiropractic adjustments often result in a pleasant sensation during the release of pressure and an overall feeling of well-being. Often, the patient will hear a "click" from the procedure.

The number of chiropractic appointments needed for treatment of menstrual problems is determined by the cause of misalignment. When simple muscle spasm is the culprit, one appointment may be all that is needed. When complicated conditions are affecting several spinal disks and joints, however, longer treatment is required, perhaps as many as three appointments each week for several months or longer.

Although chiropractic is an excellent form of therapy for musculoskeletal conditions experienced during menstruation, there are several types of disorders for which it is inappropriate, including bone infection and cancer. In addition, if you have atherosclerosis or other problems with the arteries, manipulation of the neck and lower back should be avoided.

There are many other natural healing therapies that complement chiropractic treatment, including acupuncture, aromatherapy, hatha-yoga, herbs, massage, meditation, and psychotherapy.

HATHA-YOGA

Yoga is based on the ancient Indian traditional belief that five "sheaths" of being are found in life. Imbalance of these sheaths—which include physical, mental, and spiritual energies and thought—can result in disease. Premenstrual and menstrual symptoms are seen as the manifestations of excess energies being released. Treatment for excess energies involves practicing asanas (positions) daily throughout the month. (See Chapter Three for the following exercises.) For maximum effectiveness, first perform the belly-breathing practice (see "Breathing for Relaxation") and the practice meditation (see "Meditation"), then warm up with the sun salutation (see "Hatha-Yoga"). Beginning two days before premenstrual symptoms are expected to begin, practice the relaxation imagery technique (see "Imagery") for fifteen minutes, three times a day. Continue for as many days as menstrual comfort persists.

Asanas listed below can be helpful for relieving specific menstrual discomforts. Use them when symptoms develop and continue using them until symptoms subside. Unless otherwise noted, most stretches should be held for only ten seconds initially. Gradually increase to two or even several minutes if it is comfortable.

Yoga is safe and effective and can also be used in conjunction with any other natural therapy. Some positions may exacerbate conditions like hypertension and hernia, however. Be sure to take note of any precautions listed below for individual asanas.

For General Premenstrual Symptoms of Tension and Pain

Triangle. Stand with the feet between two and three feet apart. Inhale, raising your arms parallel to the floor. Turn your right foot ninety degrees and your left foot slightly to the right. Exhale, and bend your body at the trunk to the right, while, without leaning forward, you slide your right hand down your leg toward your foot. Simultaneously raise your left arm toward the sky, palm facing forward. Look up at the left hand. Hold the position for ten to thirty seconds, breathing normally and stretching further upon each exhalation. Return to the starting position as you inhale. Repeat for the left side.

Child's Pose. This position relaxes the entire body and stretches the spine. Kneel on the floor. Slowly bring your chest as close to your knees as possible, letting your buttocks sink into your calves. Drop your forehead as close to the floor as possible. Lay arms beside your body, palms up. Hold the position for several minutes. As you become more flexible, you will be able to drop forehead farther to the floor.

Spinal Twist. This stretches and strengthens the back, which can help improve blood flow to the pelvic area. Sit with your right leg straight in front of you. Bend your left knee and place your left foot flat on floor. Lift your chest and, from your abdomen, twist to your left. For support, place your left hand on the floor behind your hips and your right elbow on the outside of your left knee. Hold the position for thirty seconds at first, gradually increasing to two minutes. Repeat the entire exercise to stretch the other side of your body.

Bow. Lie face down on your stomach. Bend your knees and bring them and your ankles toward your buttocks. Grasp your legs at the ankles, one at a time. Lift your knees off the floor by pulling the ankles away, but not down, from the hands. At the same time, lift your head up, as if the top of your head is being pulled from the top with a string. Your chest and thighs should also be off of the floor. Feel the arch along your back, like a drawn bow. Hold the position for at least ten seconds, increasing gradually to one minute.

Note: Avoid this position if you are experiencing headaches.

Corpse. Lie on the floor. Reduce the gap beneath your lower back by lifting your knees to your chest on your back, then slide your feet along the floor as you lower your legs. Spread your feet about one foot apart. Spread your arms so that they are at forty-five-degree angle from the body, with palms up. Lift your head and lower it with your chin tucked in, or rest your head on its side. Hold this position for three minutes. You can also combine this with the relaxation imagery technique described in Chapter Three.

For Painful Breasts

Camel. Kneel on the floor in an upright position—without sitting on your calves. Push your stomach out, and arch your back as you lean your head and neck backward. Drop your arms to the floor, and touch your palms to your heels by first twisting to the right and making contact with your heel, then to the right. If you can't bend back far enough to touch your heels, go as far back as possible and increase extension over time. Hold the position for ten seconds. Relax by sitting back on your heels. Repeat twice more. Gradually increase to one minute.

HERBS

Herbs make a wonderful ally in the struggle with menstrual problems, not only because they are gentler than drugs, but because they have unique healing properties not found in drugs. While many women have difficulty using the latter because of their powerful side effects, herbs restore the body and mind without overpowering either.

Herbs that have estrogenlike properties can quell menstrual complaints by providing a natural replacement therapy. Other herbs can relieve pain and discomfort with their analgesic and antispasmodic effects.

Taking the herbs below in the recommended quantities should produce results almost immediately. Once results are achieved, stop taking the herb. In all cases, do *not* take the herb for longer periods or for greater doses than recommended below. You should consult with your health professional before undertaking any herbal treatment. Herbal therapy should not be used as a substitute for standard medical care for any serious illness or infection.

Healing herbs should not be taken while using aromatherapy or homeopathy, but can be combined with most other natural therapies. For more information on herbs, see "Herbs," Chapter Three.

Black Haw (*Viburnum prunifolium*). The bark of this Native American shrub, from the same family as the honeysuckle flower, has a jaded past. An effective uterine relaxant, black haw was given to enslaved black women by their profit-minded owners to prevent miscarriage. Today, black haw is not considered safe for pregnant women, but is used widely to calm menstrual cramps by American herbalists and by German practitioners. Preparations made with black haw are widely available in Germany.

Precautions: Pregnant women should avoid black haw because it contains salicin, a chemical similar to aspirin, which has been linked with birth defects.

Preparation: For a decoction, add one and one-half teaspoons of dried bark to one cup of water. Boil for fifteen minutes. Drink no more than five cups per day. In a tincture, consume up to one teaspoonful five times per day. Black haw is available in commercial teas at your local health-food store.

Black Cohosh (*Cimicifuga racemosa* or *Macrotys actaeoides*). The roots of this plant, a member of the same family as the buttercup flower, were used by Native Americans and colonialists as a gynecological remedy. Black cohosh was also one of the main ingredients in the popular early remedy called Lydia Pinkham's vegetable compound. (A compound available today by the same name lacks the cohosh.) This herb can relieve menstrual and menopausal discomfort by mimicking the female hormone, estrogen. Decreased levels of the hormone estrogen prior to and during menstruation are believed to cause overall pain and discomfort. This herb is not available in China, but a similar herb is used for gynecological problems there. Black cohosh is also used in homeopathic remedies to treat gynecological problems.

Precautions: Because of possible side effects, this herb should be used only under the supervision of a physician. Estrogen may also contribute to liver problems and abnormal blood clotting or inflammation of blood vessels. Pregnant women should avoid black cohosh. In addition, in very large doses, black cohosh may cause side effects of subdued heart rate, dizziness, diarrhea, or abdominal pain. Thus, black cohosh should be avoided by people with heart disease and those taking sedatives or blood-pressure medication.

Preparation: For a decoction, boil one-half teaspoon of powdered root per cup of water for twenty to twenty-five minutes. Drink no more than one cup per day.

Buchu (*Barosma betulina, crenulate*, or *serratifolia*). The leaves of this five-foot native shrub of South Africa were used to cure urinary problems by indigenous people long before Europeans settled there. Buchu contains an oil that increases urine production and is used today by herbalists and in American pharmaceuticals for relief of premenstrual bloating.

Precautions: Diuretics deplete the body's store of potassium, a mineral that is vital to cell functioning. Anyone taking buchu should consume foods high in potassium, which include bananas, potatoes, and oranges. Pregnant women should avoid buchu.

Preparation: For an infusion, use one to two teaspoons of dried leaves per cup of boiling water. Steep ten to twenty minutes. Drink up to three cups per day. For a tincture, take one-half to one teaspoonful up to three times per day. Buchu tea is also available commercially at your local health-food store.

Feverfew (*Matricaria* or *Chrysanthemum parthenium*).   Most of the news that has been spread about the leaves of this plant, a member of the same family as the daisy and the dandelion, concerns its remarkable effectiveness in suppressing migraine headaches. But menstrual sufferers are the first to praise its antispasmodic effect, which causes the smooth muscles that line the uterine wall to relax. Feverfew is also believed to neutralize "bad" prostaglandins, the hormonelike chemicals in the body that are believed to play a role in causing menstrual cramps. For more information, see "Herbs," Chapter Three.

Motherwort (*Leonurus cardiaca*).   The prized leaves, flowers, and stems of this member of the mint family can be quite useful for menstrual problems for several reasons. Motherwort may be unique—rarely does an herb known to be a uterine stimulant also have a tranquilizing effect. Because of its ability to promote menstruation, it is useful for regulating the menstrual cycle, and its tranquilizing effect can be very helpful in soothing the ills related to menstruation, from anxiety to insomnia.

Precautions: Because motherwort is a uterine stimulant, it should be *avoided* by pregnant women. Because it may have anticlotting effects, it should be avoided by hemophiliacs or other people with clotting disorders. It should also be avoided by those who are taking antihypertensive, cardiac, or sedative medications. Do not give this herb to children or elderly people. Pregnant women should avoid this herb.

Preparation: For an infusion, steep two teaspoons in one cup of boiling water for fifteen minutes. Drink no more than one and one-half cups each day. In a tincture, ingest one teaspoon no more than twice each day.

Red Clover (*Trifolium pratense*). While it has been touted for a century as a cancer treatment, the flower tops of this three-leafed herb have another treasured effect. Menstrual and menopausal discomfort can be relieved by this herb's estrogenlike effects.

Precautions: Because of its estrogenlike effects, all of the same general precautions apply to using red clover as they do to black cohosh (see above). Do not give this herb to children or elderly people. Pregnant women should avoid it.

Preparation: Use two teaspoons per one cup of boiling water. Steep ten to fifteen minutes. Drink no more than four cups per day. For a tincture, use one teaspoonful no more than three times per day.

Uva Ursi (*Arctostaphylos uva-ursi*). Generations of families have used the leaves of this plant, a member of the same family as the rhododendron, as an antiseptic for healing urinary tract infections. Because of its diuretic qualities, this herb has gained favor among menstrual sufferers seeking relief from bloating and fluid retention. For more information, see "Cystitis," Chapter Five.

Vervain or Blue Vervain (*Verbena hastata*). An encyclopedic array of uses of this aspirinlike herb from the time
of the ancient Egyptians, Greeks, and Romans to the present make its leaves, flowers, and roots cherished. A species
of this is available in Europe, cousin to that available in the
United States. An anti-inflammatory agent and pain reliever, this herb can be useful for relieving a variety of
minor discomforts related to menstruation, from headache
to achiness. It also may have the ability to promote menstruation, thus making it useful for regulating the menstrual cycle. Vervain also has a mild laxative effect. For
more information, see Herbs (for "Osteoarthritis"), Chapter Nine.

HOMEOPATHY

Homeopathy's popularity with women goes back to the
beginning of its development. Today it is a favorite with
men as well and gets its fame as the medicine of choice of
England's royal family. Homeopathic remedies are helpful
in managing menstrual problems because remedies are
based on substances that would stimulate symptoms of
menstruation in a non-sufferer. Unlike drugs that combat
symptoms at the expense of thwarting the body's attempt
to become well, homeopathic remedies activate the body's
natural defenses for relieving pain and discomfort. And if
you use homeopathic treatments regularly, you will become less susceptible to developing symptoms in the first
place.

Because the characteristics of homeopathic remedies
must be closely matched to an individual's personality and
idiosyncracies before becoming effective, it's important to
match your feelings and physical symptoms as closely as
possible with the remedies listed below, just as a homeo-

path would. Unless otherwise noted, take a dose of 30c. For premenstrual discomfort, take remedies twice each day for up to three days, beginning twenty-four hours before symptoms typically start. For menstrual discomfort, take the remedy every hour for up to ten doses as soon as menstrual cramps begin. In both cases, *stop* taking medication once symptoms begin to improve. If your medication has no effect, it usually indicates that you have taken the wrong remedy. In that case, review your symptoms, and, being as specific as possible, match them to another remedy.

Homeopathic formulations will not interfere with the action of prescription drugs. However, some drugs may block the effects of homeopathic remedies, at least to some degree. They include steroids, tranquilizers, birth control pills, sleeping pills, and antihistamines. Do *not* stop taking drugs prescribed by your physician without first consulting him or her. Homeopathy may be used in conjunction with some therapies like acupuncture, chiropractic, and hypnosis (Chapter Eight) or psychotherapy. But it should not generally be used simultaneously with aromatherapy or herbs because the former's essential oils may inactivate the homeopathic solution, as will coffee, alcohol, tobacco, perfumed cosmetics, and pungent household cleansers. Before taking any remedy, you should also consult with an appropriate health professional.

To Relieve Premenstrual Symptoms

- *Calcarea carbonica:* Use this to pep up when feeling exhausted or sluggish. It also helps to minimize breast tenderness, cold sweats, and possibly "sweet tooth" cravings.

- *Causticum:* This remedy is twofold: it combats feelings of gloom and irritability, or "touchiness," and it alleviates symptoms of a mild cystitis like pains in the lower abdomen and the frequent urge to urinate.

- *Kali carbonicum:* This is a good tension reliever and is especially effective for overweight people.

- *Lachesis:* Use this remedy when symptoms are worse in the morning and for breast tenderness.

- *Lycopodium clavatum:* Try this for relief of low-blood-sugar symptoms such as feeling angry or depressed or craving sweets.

- *Natrum muriaticum:* This remedy can help to relieve the very common premenstrual symptom of swelling in the legs, feet, and breasts. It will also tend to minimize emotional irritability and sadness.

- *Nux vomica:* Use this to cure a variety of complaints: irritability, chills, frequent urination, constipation, craving sweet or fatty foods.

- *Pulsatilla:* This should help to regulate periods. It will also help if you feel sad and weepy and your breasts are tender.

- *Sepia:* Try this remedy if you're feeling irritable, chilly, weepy, emotionally lethargic, crave sweet or salty foods, or experience a diminished libido.

- *Sulphur:* This provides relief of low-blood-sugar symptoms, particularly "sweet tooth" cravings.

For Menstrual Discomfort
or Irregular Menstruation

- *Belladonna:* When you feel sharp pains that are aggravated by movement and are flushed and congested, this remedy will often bring great relief.

- *Chamomile:* Try this to subdue negative emotional symptoms like irritability or outrage and severe menstrual cramps that feel like muscle spasms.

- *Cimicifuga:* When nervousness and restlessness or dejection are combined with laborlike pains, this can help tremendously.

- *Conium maculatum:* When breasts are very sore, either before and during periods, this may bring great relief.

- *Gelsemium sempervirens:* Headaches and heavy cramps may be relieved with this wonderful remedy.

- *Hamemelis virginica:* Try this to alleviate bleeding between menstrual periods. Note: such bleeding could be a warning sign that another, more serious condition has developed (see Chapter Five and Chapter Eight).

- *Lac caninum:* If your breasts are swollen and sore, you sometimes feel dizzy, and have emotional symptoms of irritability and rage, this remedy may be of help.

- *Sabina:* When menstrual period comes early and very heavy, this will help to "right" your cycle. Note: this condition could be a warning sign that another, more serious condition has developed (see Chapter Five and Chapter Eight).

- *Urtica urens:* For extra heavy and sustained periods, this will help to restore regularity. Note: this condition could be a warning sign that another, more serious condition has developed (see Chapter Five and Chapter Eight).

For Pain During Ovulation

- *Colocynthis:* If you get some relief from pressing your lower abdomen, and you feel irate and touchy, this remedy will often provide relief. Sometimes the abdominal pain is worse on left side.

For Depression Only, Without Physical Symptoms

- Take 6c of *Pulsatilla,* listed above. *Nux vomica* or *Sepia,* also listed above, can be considered as well, depending on which remedy more closely matches your emotional symptoms.

HYDROTHERAPY

The penetrating effects of water can have therapeutic effects on the entire body, including the nervous system, the muscles, and the liver. Cryogenic (cold) and heat therapies form an integral part of hydrotherapy, which is based on the principle that treating one part of the body will affect another or several parts. There are many time-tested applications listed below that are useful to soothe the ills experienced during the menstrual cycle. For example, the sitz bath, which relieves pelvic pain, is one of the oldest hydrotherapy techniques known. Hydrotherapy draws on the therapeutic effects of warm or hot water, which is essentially relaxing, and cold water, which is predominately restorative and revitalizing.

For Premenstrual or Menstrual Cramps and Pelvic Pain

A sitz bath, or sitting bath, is an easy and practical way of treating pelvic conditions. The contemporary sitz bath is made so that a person may sit inside it comfortably while her feet rest outside in a footbath. A hot sitz bath (105 to 110 degrees Fahrenheit) is used to treat pelvic pain during the menstrual cycle and for pelvic inflammatory conditions.

To create a makeshift sitz bath, you will need two containers, one of which is large enough to sit in with ample space left over for water. A smaller container should accommodate the feet. Fill the large container with hot but not scalding water, so that water covers the pelvic area up to the navel. Fill a second container with enough hot water to cover the feet. If you cannot find suitable containers, you can simulate a sitz bath in your bathtub by pulling the knees in so that only the pelvic area and feet are covered by water. Immerse in the tub immediately, so cooling does not take place. Sit comfortably for fifteen minutes, and you'll soon feel the soothing effects. For maximum effect, top off containers with additional hot water.

A hot, moist compress on the abdomen can have an antispasmodic effect; that is, it can relax muscles that line the uterus and often contract to cause pain. Saturate a towel with hot but not scalding water. Wring out excessive moisture and fold in half. Lie down, and place the towel immediately over the lower abdomen for about ten to fifteen minutes. To maximize effectiveness, keep a bowl of very hot water at your bedside to refresh the compress every five minutes. A variation on this technique, called a fomentation, utilizes a wool-blanket material that is lined with a cotton material (a sheet, perhaps) to retain both moisture and heat. Follow the same instructions for a compress, but immerse the cotton in hot water. Then cover with the dry, wool material. Protect the bony areas of the body by lifting the fomentation occasionally to allow steam to escape.

For Diuretic or Laxative Effect

A hot, moist compress (see above), when used on the lower back, can minimize bloating caused by excessive fluid retention by stimulating the kidneys to increase urine production. Alternating a hot compress with a cold one can also have the same effect. Drinking ice water can also promote a diuretic response, as well as have a mild laxative effect.

To Relieve Insomnia

Besides relieving pain, a fomentation (see above) can have a sedative effect. Follow the same instructions above, but lay the cotton-wool material across the length of the spine for at least twenty minutes before bedtime. It should induce a restful sleep.

Hot and warm baths also have a soothing effect. For relaxation and to encourage deep sleep, submerge in warm or hot water up to your neck for twenty minutes before bedtime.

Precautions: Don't use very hot baths if you have kidney or cardiovascular conditions without first checking with your physician.

To Relieve Fatigue

See "Hydrotherapy," Chapter Three.

IMAGERY

A wide imagination and your own meaningful experiences are the only tools you'll need to promote healing with the safe and effective therapy of imagery. Imagery taps into the mind's eye to minimize our response to stress, and it can reduce the symptoms of disease. If you are feeling the pain and discomfort of menstruation, you can promote improvement by visualizing your recovery, which, in turn, can reduce symptoms. Imagery may also be helpful during the menstrual cycle because it can help to relieve the depression or anxiety that are believed to heighten menstrual discomfort. Try the relaxation imagery technique (see "Imagery," Chapter Three) twice daily to relax. If you are experiencing great pain, adapt the exercise to include some very stimulating images, or develop a scene in which your uterus is becoming relaxed and open, so that blood can flow without resistance. Don't forget to make the images as detailed and meaningful as possible to enhance imagery's effectiveness.

Imagery can be used in conjunction with any natural therapy but offers its greatest advantages when combined with biofeedback (Chapter Two), hypnosis (Chapter Eight), and other relaxation techniques.

MASSAGE

As you learned in Chapter Three, massage is a door not only to a relaxed emotional state, but also to a keen awareness of the five senses. A wide array of massage techniques can be used to invigorate or relax us, restoring balance between mind and body. Massage increases circulation in the entire body and relieves emotional tension that can become manifested in the muscles. Massage therapy has a wide variety of applications for relieving menstrual cramping.

The following techniques may be used to relieve menstrual pain. Ask a friend to read the instructions and apply these natural techniques. The Massage Warmup (see "Massage," Chapter Three) will increase circulation in the entire body, including in the pelvic area, where thwarted blood flow may contribute to cramping. In addition, the full-body massage will soothe and also loosen tissue, thus making individual applications more effective.

Massage can be used in conjunction with any alternative therapy, and is often combined with acupressure, aromatherapy, and chiropractic. For additional applications using essential oils, see "Aromatherapy," Chapter Three.

General Premenstrual and Menstrual Symptoms of Discomfort

The nerves in the sacral region, the lowest part of the spine, near the buttocks, are linked to the reproductive organs and, when irritated, they can contribute to menstrual discomfort. They are enmeshed in the sacral bone, so pressing on this bone can relieve irritations. While lying on your side, ask your helper to put one hand on the lower abdomen. With the other hand, rub about six-inch circles on the sacrum in a counterclockwise direction. Be sure to apply appropriate pressure—press firmly, but not enough to cause pain. Now repeat the same exercise, but on the lower back instead of the sacrum. Now alternate rubbing the lower back and sacral area, while still keeping one hand on the abdomen.

Lie on your stomach. Your helper should be on his or her knees, which are straddled on both sides of your body. She or he should place one hand on each side of the lumbar spine (just above the sacrum). Feel a slight impression about an inch away from the spine on each side. With the thumbs, rub in a small circular motion gently for about two minutes. Now work down the spine, inch by inch, rubbing each area until the end is reached.

Lie on the floor and place a book beneath the buttocks. Lay your hands on your lower abdomen, about half the distance between the hips and the vulva. Feel for a small hollow on each side of the abdomen. Rub in a small circular motion gently for about two to three minutes. This is a good quick-relief technique for pain, perhaps during the several hours when menstrual cramps are at a peak.

Lie on your back. Your helper should squat down with one leg on each side of your thighs and put one hand on each hip. She or he should lift your left hip slightly in the air while holding your right hip securely. Allow the left hip to sink to the floor while raising the right hip. Rock the hips like this for two to three minutes. It will release the tension in the pelvic area.

MEDITATION

Meditation is an excellent therapy for women with menstrual problems because it allows you to relax and experience peace and tranquility. While other therapies promote a certain therapeutic physical response, meditation produces a state of mind that is therapeutic in that anxiety and depression are reduced, thus relieving the menstrual discomfort that can become magnified as a result of such emotions. Disturbing thoughts are observed but are felt to be secondary to a state of quiet existence. When you experience menstrual symptoms, you may feel anxious because of the problems they cause in your life, either at home or at work. Meditation gives you an opportunity to focus away from these anxieties and quiet the mind. Besides ameliorating the symptoms of menstruation, meditation is effective in reducing susceptibility to a host of stress-related illnesses and conditions. Try the practice meditation (see "Meditation," Chapter Three) twice daily to relax. If you are experiencing great pain, try to observe anxious thoughts that accompany pain and let go of them. You may find that daily meditation not only helps to quell menstrual problems, but changes your outlook on life!

Meditation can be combined with virtually any natural therapy.

NUTRITIONAL THERAPY

Deficiencies of certain nutrients have been linked with menstrual problems, and, in general, the diets of those with such problems dramatically differ from those without symptoms. According to several studies, the diets of premenstrual sufferers tend to be much higher in refined carbohydrates and sugars and dairy products than the diets of the symptom-free. Results of a typical study of premenstrual sufferers are shown below. Percentages of foods consumed, compared to those of the symptom-free, are given:

- 275 percent more refined sugar
- 79 percent more dairy products
- 78 percent more sodium
- 62 percent more refined carbohydrates (e.g., bleached flour)
- 53 percent less iron

- 77 percent less manganese
- 52 percent less zinc.

Unless you constantly opt for "junk" and empty-calorie foods over a nutritious meal, you're probably not contributing greatly to your menstrual discomforts. If, however, the above list looks quite familiar—that is, you eat a lot of foods high in salt, sugar, and bleached flour; a lot of dairy products; and very few whole-grain foods, fresh fruits, or vegetables, you are no doubt contributing to menstrual discomfort as well as depriving your body of valuable vitamins and minerals.

Minerals

Minerals are essential to almost every body process. They transport oxygen to each cell, regulate the heartbeat, maintain proper fluid and chemical balances, and form components of hormones. Minerals are usually interdependent—that is, an imbalance in one mineral usually results in an imbalance in another. Calcium, magnesium, and phosphorus are called the major minerals because they are most abundant in the body.

Magnesium plays a vital role in preventing menstrual symptoms. It is needed for the synthesis of sex hormones, including estrogen, the levels of which are lowered during menstruation. Magnesium is necessary for proper muscle and nerve function. Without enough magnesium, we become worn down and supersensitive to pain. Common menstrual symptoms—nervousness, breast tenderness, irritability, anxiety, and weight gain—are often the result. A magnesium deficiency can result from stress, the use of diuretics, and high quantities of refined sugar in the diet, which causes the kidney to increase excretion of magnesium. Thus, when premenstrual sufferers consume foods that are high in refined sugar, they are laying the groundwork for a magnesium deficiency.

Calcium, the body's most plentiful mineral, can also contribute to a magnesium deficiency when levels exceed the normal ratio with magnesium. Calcium makes up about one and one-half to two pounds of a woman's body, mostly in the bones and teeth. A small percentage of calcium functions as a nerve and muscle relaxant and contributes to other essential body processes. Very great deficiencies of calcium may contribute to menstrual symptoms. However, calcium's most important role in menarche is its regulation of other minerals, like magnesium.

When we consume too much calcium from a diet high in dairy products, we are contributing to a magnesium deficiency. Too much calcium can also be caused by the presence of the "bad" prostaglandins, hormonelike chemicals that increase this mineral's uptake in the body (see below).

Thus, when premenstrual sufferers typically consume foods high in dairy products *and* refined sugar, they are in effect contributing to a chronic magnesium deficiency, which produces menstrual symptoms.

B-Complex Vitamins

Called the "energy" vitamins, the eight B vitamins that make up the B complex are essential for nerve and muscle functions. A deficiency of these vitamins is said to be linked with menstrual cramping, excessive menstrual bleeding, and fibrocystic breast disease (see Chapter Five). Most instrumental in the menstrual process is vitamin B_6 (pyridoxine), which regulates the chemical balance in the tissues and excretion of water, and helps regulate muscle, lymph, nerve, and liver processes. Vitamin B_6 helps to relieve menstrual symptoms by facilitating the absorption of magnesium and inhibiting the secretion of prolactin, the hormone that stimulates the mammary glands in the breast. Excessive levels of prolactin have been found in blood levels of premenstrual women with extremely tender breasts. Thus, a deficiency of vitamin B_6 can lead to breast soreness, as well as exacerbate mood changes and cause headaches.

"Good" and "Bad" Prostaglandins

It seems like every metabolic process in the body has its bad influences and good influences, and menstruation is no different. Hormonelike substances called prostaglandins battle it out to regulate physiological processes that occur in the body including menstruation, and conditions from high blood pressure to tumor growth. High levels of the "bad" prostaglandins can cause all of the undesirable symptoms associated with the menstrual cycle—fluid retention, breast tenderness, "hungry horrors" including the "sweet tooth" variety, fatigue, dizziness, and even heart palpitations. The "good" prostaglandins, of course, try to intercede and counteract all of those heinous symptoms. They can inhibit the extra secretion of insulin that lowers blood sugar and causes food cravings, dizziness, and fatigue. The trouble arises when the "good" prostaglandins are outnumbered by the "bad" prostaglandins. Whichever substance bands in the greatest numbers, of course, wins. So, one key to promoting a tolerable menstrual period is to encourage synthesis of the "good" prostaglandins. In order for the body to synthesize these "good" substances, it needs adequate amounts of—yes—vitamin B_6 and magnesium, as well as zinc, vitamin C and vitamin B_3 (niacin). Gamma-linolenic acid (GLA), found in some plants (see "Nutritional Therapy," Chapter Three) and in evening-primrose oil (see below), is also needed to synthesize the "good" prostaglandins. Like many other nutrients, GLA cannot be synthesized without the presence of adequate levels of—you guessed it—magnesium and vitamin B_6, as well as zinc and vitamin C. It's important to note that GLA synthesis can be suppressed by a diet high in cholesterol, trans-fatty acids (from hydrogenated vegetable oils like margarine), refined sugar, and alcohol. Stress can also inhibit GLA synthesis.

Eating Healthfully

To put it simply, the body can only work with the foods you consume. If you are eating poorly, you are not giving it much to work with and are no doubt exacerbating not only menstrual symptoms, but inhibiting other physiological processes as well. It's best to stick with dietary sources to obtain needed nutrients. (For a list of nutritional sources, see "Nutritional Therapy," Chapter Three.) The body absorbs vitamins and minerals from food sources more easily than it does those found in supplements. And when given nutrient-rich foods, the body does a marvelous balancing act—it will retain more of a nutrient from foods if levels are low, and less if stores are sufficient or too high.

If you're like the premenstrual sufferer in the study above, you should reduce consumption of dairy products. Calcium is very important in the development and maintenance of bone health, however, so be sure to consume *at least* the recommended dietary allowance of 1,000 milligrams per day! (Many nutritionists think that the U.S. dietary allowance of 800 milligrams is too low for women's needs.)

To minimize fluid retention and swelling, cut back on salt and high-sodium foods. Try naturally diuretic foods such as cranberry juice, watermelon, cucumber, asparagus, parsley, and strawberries, which are useful if eaten alone.

Coffee, tea, and chocolate, which also promote diuretic action, contain substances that may contribute to menstrual problems. These substances cause short bursts of energy that lead to an overall tired feeling and promote muscle contractions that can contribute to cramps.

To enhance the synthesis of the body's natural painkilling hormones that can be activated by acupressure, acupuncture, and aerobic exercise, adequate levels of tryptophan, an essential amino acid, as well as vitamins C, B_6, and B_{12}, are necessary. Tryptophan, which is found in many protein-rich foods, is absorbed in the body only after meals containing carbohydrates. Thus, the easiest way to increase tryptophan levels is to sprinkle a moderate amount of cheese on pasta, potatoes, or other carbohydrates.

Keep in mind, however, that most nutritional remedies for menstruation take from one to three months before improvements are felt.

Vitamin Supplements

If you are clearly unable to provide yourself with adequate food sources of a particular nutrient (e.g., you're a vegetarian, or you live in a climate where some important foods are unavailable), taking a vitamin supplement can be very helpful. Included in the vitamin supplement should be the B-complex vitamins (all eight), because a surplus of one B vitamin may lead to a deficiency in another. Some nutritionists recommend taking B-complex vitamins plus a vitamin B_6 supplement. If you decide to do this, limit the B_6 dose to 50 milligrams, morning and night, beginning three days before you expect premenstrual symptoms. Continue until your menstrual period begins. You can take the B-complex vitamins every day until symptoms subside.

Precautions: High doses of vitamin B_6 (250 milligrams

per day) can lead to neurological problems. Also, most reactions to vitamins result from taking them on an empty
stomach. Vitamins should be taken with meals for better
digestion and absorption.

A proper B-complex vitamin pill will contain the ratios
listed below. Be sure to check the label. Some manufacturers cut costs by supplying more than is needed of the least
expensive vitamins and less than needed of others.

Vitamin	Milligrams
B_1 (thiamine)	50
B_2 (riboflavin)	50
B_3 (niacin)	150
B_6 (pyridoxine)	100
B_{12} (cobalamin)	200
Folic acid (folacin)	400
Biotin	200
Pantothenic acid	100

Bioactive Supplements

Bioactive supplements, now available in the U.S. market,
are a healthier alternative to traditional vitamin supplements. Bioactive supplements, which include algae and
pollen, are whole foods and are easily recognized and absorbed by the body. Vitamin supplements, on the other
hand, contain isolated and synthetic chemicals that may
promote attacks by the body's immune system.

Bioactive supplements can be helpful in preventing and
treating a range of women's health concerns including
menstrual-related problems. Two types of algae called
spirulina and chlorella are now available in health food
stores; both contain a wide range of nutrients—from

B-vitamins to minerals and high-grade protein. Spirulina also offers an abundant source of iron.

Evening-Primrose Oil

A favorite remedy for menstrual sufferers, evening-primrose oil is made from the seeds of the evening primrose flower. It's very effective in lowering blood cholesterol and blood pressure, but menstrual-period sufferers have long noted its healing effect for conditions such as breast tenderness and cramps. Evening-primrose oil is high in gamma-linolenic acid (GLA), which helps to synthesize "good" prostaglandins that minimize menstrual symptoms. Evening-primrose oil may also inhibit the release of the hormone prolactin, which activates the mammary glands and is believed to be responsible for symptoms of breast swelling and tenderness during premenstruation. It is available in capsules at your local health-food store. Two capsules, one in the morning and one at night, are recommended for menstrual problems. Possible side effects include headaches and a feeling of lethargy. If you experience these symptoms, discontinue use.

PSYCHOTHERAPY

Women who suffer from severe menstrual discomfort often find that the emotional symptoms—irritability, anger, or depression—are the most difficult to handle. While these symptoms can be somewhat subdued by the various therapies described here, often there is a limit to the level of comfort that can be attained. Thus, learning to manage the challenges of emotional duress is a task faced by millions of American women. Symptoms can be heightened even further when the emotional tumult leads to conflicts in the office or at home. This can produce a "secondary" anxiety, a fear that menstrual symptoms will heighten or present problems in our lives. Besides intensifying menstrual symptoms, this secondary anxiety obviously makes our lives harder to live during these particular days or weeks of the month.

Thus, psychotherapy can be a valuable tool for menstrual sufferers to explore ways to handle the emotional stress. It also provides an avenue to validate the suffering felt during the menstrual cycle. Menstruation is, in fact, a complex biochemical process that dramatically alters the hormonal balance of women's bodies and thus can strongly affect our moods. Our symptoms can be influenced by a range of lifestyle factors, including diet, exercise, emotional health, social support, and stress.

Of course, menstrual problems are influenced by emotional factors, so women who are depressed or anxious may find that symptoms of discomfort are intensified. These emotional states are often present not just during menstruation, but other times as well. Thus, if you are prone to psychological symptoms of depression or great anxiety during menstruation or all month, you may benefit from consulting with a psychotherapist.

Alleviating the sources of stress that contribute to menstrual problems seems to be an obvious and direct solution, but realistically this is not always possible nor even recommended on short notice. Deciding to get a divorce or relocate, for example, are major changes that require great introspection and thought, a process for which psychotherapy can be helpful. Psychotherapy can also be helpful in zeroing in on the sources of stress that may contribute to menstrual problems, sources that are often mistakenly trivialized in terms of their effect on our lives and health. Psychotherapy can help us to successfully cope with these stresses. Even changes for the better can produce stress. If, on the other hand, your frustrations are based on minor annoyances, incorporating simple relaxation exercises into your life may be helpful (see "Breathing for Relaxation," Chapter Three). In either case, learning relaxation techniques may be helpful in reducing menstrual symptoms. Study results indicate that stress-reduction strategies, when practiced regularly, can raise the threshold of provocation before a stress response occurs.

If you decide to see a psychotherapist, she or he will evaluate your problem by discussing with you feelings and concerns, then make a recommendation about whether therapy would be beneficial and how long treatment might last. Short-term treatment could involve weekly appointments for three to six months, while long-term psychotherapy sessions may involve one to three weekly sessions for several years. Ask your psychotherapist about his or her background and training, and the type of psychotherapy practiced. Some psychotherapists strictly follow one type of therapy, while others are eclectic and employ a variety of therapeutic techniques. (For more information about forms of therapy, see Chapter Two.)

Psychotherapy can be used with virtually any other alternative therapy, and when combined with mind-body therapies like biofeedback (Chapter Two); breathing for relaxation, hatha-yoga, and hypnosis (Chapter Eight); and meditation can produce powerful results. Besides promoting relaxation, the latter therapies can heighten personal insight.

CHAPTER FIVE

Pelvic Infections and Benign Gynecological Concerns

Today, several women's health conditions are increasingly of concern. Breast lumps affect at least one in four women. So do uterine lumps. Endometriosis, called the "career woman's disease," now affects as many as 9 million women. Bladder infections (cystitis) and vaginal infections (vaginitis) recur with such extraordinary frequency that the latter is estimated to account for one in ten visits to the gynecologist!

What all of these conditions have in common is their ability to be affected by a woman's lifestyle. Emotional and psychological factors, for example, can contribute to the development of these conditions. Just as emotional tension can become lodged in the muscles and interfere with functioning, so can it become trapped in the reproductive organs and lead to physiological dysfunction. A uterine problem like endometriosis or fibroid lumps is sometimes influenced by issues of sexuality or womanhood. Women with these problems may be suppressing feelings of anxiety or confusion about sexuality, anger against a partner, or mistrust arising from experience of sexual abuse, for example. Because the breast typically symbolizes nurturing, a history of emotional neglect or overprotection during childhood may result in an energy imbalance that develops into breast-related conditions in adulthood.

Benign conditions may also be affected by environmental factors. Numerous toxins that enter our body each day from food and environmental sources are filtered from the blood by the body's liver. The liver is also responsible for the breakdown of estrogen to make it available for use by the body. Thus, when toxins overload the liver, it becomes overworked and is unable to perform all of its jobs, including the breakdown of estrogen, efficiently. Excessive levels of estrogen cannot be released by the body until they are metabolized by the liver, so they circulate and eventually build up, and are believed to contribute to the development of conditions like breast and uterine lumps and endometriosis.

Cystitis and vaginitis are other increasingly common conditions that are influenced by lifestyle factors. Many Americans are eating proportionately higher amounts of refined sugars and carbohydrates, which upset the balance in the body, including the vagina. Because infections can be passed back and forth between partners, increased sexual freedom may contribute to the high recurrence rate of vaginitis and cystitis. But, ironically, the number one cause of vaginitis is allopathic antibiotics developed to treat cystitis! Drugs intended to kill bacteria in the bladder also offset the balance of microorganisms in the vagina, making it vulnerable to infection. Other allopathic treatment for infection and benign conditions can sometimes do more harm than good. Medicated creams prescribed for vaginitis, like drugs, throw off the natural balance of the body. Allopathic treatment for breast and uterine lumps and endometriosis often entails surgical procedures from lumpectomy to hysterectomy. The hysterectomy has been employed for centuries as a cure-all for everything from menstrual cramps to, ironically, menopause. Given these alternatives, it's not surprising that many women are turning to natural medicine for gentler approaches to healing common health problems.

BREAST LUMPS

Most of the breast is made up of fatty tissue that surrounds a network of milk-producing bulbs and lobes arranged around the nipple. Ducts connect these lobes with the nipple. The nipple contains glands that lubricate by producing oily substances, as well as erectile tissue that causes them to stand out when stimulated, to make them accessible to the infant.

Every month after a young woman reaches puberty, the menstrual cycle will stimulate hormones that will cause changes in her breasts. The hormones estrogen and progesterone will increase blood flow to the breasts and cause them to retain more fluid. Estrogen will also cause stimulation of the milk-producing glands in the breast, causing them to become larger and more full. After these changes have taken place, menstruation will occur, and the breasts will return to their original size and makeup. In some cases, however, the extra tissue may not completely be reabsorbed before the next cycle begins. Thus, some tissue remains, and over a period of time builds up. Over time, this buildup often becomes inflamed and causes a response by the body in which it begins to break down the natural tissue, forming cysts.

Another process can contribute to breast lumps as well. Estrogen can irritate the breast because of inefficient liver production, which allows the circulating levels of estrogen in the body to build up.

Because predisposing factors to breast lumps are quite common, most women experience some kind of lumpiness in their breasts, either cysts that are fluid-filled or solid lumps called fibroadenomas, anytime from menarche to menopause. At least 80 percent of breast lumps are benign, and the majority of these benign lumps that occur are as a result of fibrocystic breast disease.

Benign breast lumps can be distinguished from malignant or cancerous lumps in several ways. Unlike benign lumps, malignant lumps do not usually cause pain. They also do not generally fluctuate in size or disappear and reoccur as benign lumps can. Finally, after menopause, most benign lumps disappear on their own.

Despite its misleading name, fibrocystic breast disease simply means that you, like 25 to 50 percent of fertile women, have lumpy, often painful breasts. Lumps are usually fluid-filled, numerous, and move around in the breast during palpation. They typically cause pain, but can be painless until surges in estrogen are highest—before the menstrual period, during pregnancy, or during surges of perimenopause. Evidence once suggested that fibrocystic breast disease was a precursor of breast cancer, but more recent evidence suggests that it is not, leaving the cancer link still unclear. Despite this, many allopathic surgeons routinely remove solid lumps in case they might develop into breast cancer some day. While precaution is certainly necessary in some circumstances—some fibroadenomas closely resemble some rare types of breast cancer—surgery can have traumatic effects on the body and the emotions. Thus, most natural practitioners recommend that natural therapies first be used to alleviate the many conditions that can contribute to the development of breast lumps.

ACUPRESSURE/ACUPUNCTURE
(FOR BREAST LUMPS)

In the ancient Eastern therapies of acupressure and acupuncture, illness results from improper energy flow in the body. In Chinese medicine, the liver meridian, which controls the breast, is usually the trouble spot that can promote breast lumps. In general, breast lumps that are movable tend to be caused by stagnant *chi,* while nonmovable masses usually result from stuck blood.

While *chi* can stagnate in several organs, the liver is the most common and usual place for stagnant *chi* to begin. However, if not dealt with, the stagnation can intensify and/or spread to other organs. Of course, because of the interdependent relationship between *chi* and blood, stagnant *chi* may result in stagnant blood or vice versa. Stuck *chi* may also be caused by injury, overeating, smoking marijuana, or stagnation of dampness caused by damp weather, working in a damp environment, disharmony of the spleen, eating foods that promote dampness, or any combination of these factors. If stagnant food or dampness continues untreated for any period of time, it may develop into phlegm, which can then form into lumps or tumors. Thus, acupuncture treatment for benign breast lumps will involve correcting these imbalances and usually includes stimulating the liver to help mobilize *chi.*

- *Liver 14:* You'll find this point two ribs below the nipple in the sixth intercostal space.
- *Small intestine 11:* This point is located inside the large hollow in the middle of the shoulder blade. You may feel a slight soreness when you touch this point because it is very sensitive.

- *Liver 3:* This point is located on the top of the foot in the depression beyond the juncture of the metatarsal bones of the big toe and the second toe.

BREATHING FOR RELAXATION (FOR BREAST LUMPS)

The breasts represent nurturing in life, and the development of breast lumps is sometimes related to emotional issues surrounding sustenance. Breast lumps can result from repressed resentment of being either overprotected or undernourished during youth. Relaxation may be especially helpful in releasing the emotional tension that may underlie breast lumps or perhaps is making them more painful. If you are feeling stressed about this issue, chances are that you are feeling the stress in other areas of your life as well. Relaxation can be helpful in relieving the stress that may be dampening your experience of life and in restoring your vitality. Learning how to breathe healthfully is the first step in managing stress because it averts the rapid, shallow breathing of the body's stress response. Try the belly-breathing practice in "Breathing for Relaxation," Chapter Three.

HATHA-YOGA (FOR BREAST/UTERINE LUMPS AND ENDOMETRIOSIS)

Although hatha-yoga stretches provide excellent physical benefits, this therapy emphasizes the spiritual aspects of being. Illness can occur when any of the five spiritual planes are offset.

Hatha-yoga slow movements can provide just the right amount of gentle stimulation for moving the energies that can become blocked or misdirected in the body's organs. Exercises promote a sense of involvement with the body, helping women to reconnect themselves with it and all of its parts—to feel whole again. Asanas can help women to appreciate their femaleness and their bodies because pleasant feelings result when women learn to work with their bodies to accomplish movements. Once blocked emotional and physical energies in the reproductive organs are released, women can celebrate their own uniqueness, rejoice in their sexuality, and regain balance in their lives.

Yoga treatment involves practicing asanas throughout the month. (See Chapter Three for the following exercises.) For maximum effectiveness, first perform the belly-breathing practice (see "Breathing for Relaxation") and the practice meditation (see "Meditation"), then warm up with the sun salutation (see "Hatha-Yoga"). Specific applications are listed below for women with breast and uterine lumps and endometriosis.

For breast lumps, the camel position is recommended (see "Hatha-Yoga," Chapter Four). For uterine lumps or endometriosis, the following are recommended:

Triangle (see "Hatha-Yoga," Chapter Four)
Child's Pose (see "Hatha-Yoga," Chapter Four)
Bow (see "Hatha-Yoga," Chapter Four)
Abdominal Rock (see "Hatha-Yoga," Chapter Seven)

HERBS (FOR BREAST/UTERINE LUMPS AND ENDOMETRIOSIS)

Herbs can provide a unique healing action not available through drugs to heal hormone-related conditions such as breast and uterine lumps and endometriosis. The first line of defense against such conditions should be herbs that

promote the functioning of the liver, because its ineffi-
ciency is most likely contributing to estrogen-related conditions. But herbs play another role in relieving hormone-
related conditions as well. Some herbs have estrogenlike
properties that may make them useful in counteracting the
effects of estrogen-dependent conditions. This is possible
because herbs supply a natural form of estrogen that is less
potent than the body's own estrogen. When provided with
these estrogenlike herbs, the body will absorb the gentler
estrogen and release the stronger estrogen from the body.
Other herbs supply a natural form of progesterone, excessive levels of which may be related to endometriosis, and
play the same beneficial role as estrogenlike herbs.

Taking the herbs below in the recommended quantities
may minimize some symptoms almost immediately, but
benefits will increase incrementally over time. In all cases,
do *not* take the herb for longer periods or in greater doses
than recommended below.

Herbs should not be taken while using aromatherapy or
homeopathy, but can be combined with most other natural
therapies. You should consult with your health professional
before undertaking herbal treatment. Herbal therapy
should not be used as a substitute for standard medical
care for any serious condition.

For more information on herbs, see "Herbs," Chapter
Three.

To Promote Liver Functioning

Milk Thistle (*Carduus marianus*).   This herb has been
used by Europeans as a method of enhancing the functioning of the liver and makes a wonderful liver-cleanser and
promoter. Milk thistle can also be helpful in promoting
liver metabolism, which is often compromised by environ-

mental or dietary factors. For more information, see "Herbs," Chapter Eight.

Turmeric (*Curcuma longa*). The roots of this member of the same family as ginger are prized by those with arthritis for their ability to reduce pain and inflammation. But women with estrogen-related difficulties may also benefit from turmeric's ability to protect the liver and promote its functioning. For more information, see Herbs (for "Osteoarthritis"), Chapter Nine.

To Relieve Excessive Estrogen Levels

Angelica (*Angelica atropurpurea*). The roots and leaves of this ancient herb have been used for centuries for everything from magic to treating malaria, but women with estrogen-related conditions may gain the most benefit from its ability to regulate the body's estrogen. Angelica works by supplying a natural and less toxic form of estrogen to the body, which is absorbed in lieu of the body's own stronger estrogen.

Precautions: Pregnant women should avoid this drug. It should not be given to children or elderly people. Avoid fresh roots because they are poisonous. Drying eliminates the danger.

Preparation: Steep one teaspoon of dried herb in a cup of boiling water for fifteen to twenty minutes. Drink no more than two cups per day.

Lady's mantle (*Alchemilla vulgaris*). The dried leaves of this popular herb, which gets its name from alchemy because of the belief that it can promote miracle cures, can be quite beneficial in reducing estrogen levels because of its estrogenlike effects. But its most notable healing action may be its ability to regulate menstruation and relieve heavy bleeding, making it a valuable tool for women with endometriosis or uterine lumps. Lady's mantle can also provide headache relief.

Precautions: Pregnant women should avoid this herb. It should not be given to children or elderly people.

Preparation: Steep one teaspoon of dried herb in a cup of boiling water for ten minutes. Drink no more than one cup per day.

IMAGERY (FOR BREAST LUMPS)

Breast lumps may appear as the result of unresolved conflicts or emotional turbulences within one's life. Relaxation imagery can soothe and revitalize the body and mind, thus lessening the pain associated with some lumps and the potential for the development of further breast problems. Try the relaxation imagery technique (see "Imagery," Chapter Three) twice daily to relax.

Imagery can be used in conjunction with any natural therapy, but offers its greatest advantages when combined with biofeedback (Chapter Two), hypnosis (Chapter Eight), and other relaxation techniques.

MEDITATION (FOR BREAST/UTERINE LUMPS AND ENDOMETRIOSIS)

Meditation provides the perfect way to remain calm while under emotional or physical stress. The purpose of meditation is to create a tranquil and soothing state of existence in which you are not required to act, and thoughts are only observed, not reacted to. In short, it's a good way of promoting your ability to remain in the present, which can enhance your ability to let go of old fears and frustrations. Mediation can also relieve painful symptoms by minimizing anxiety. Moreover, it reduces our susceptibility to stress-related illnesses. Try the practice meditation (see "Meditation," Chapter Three) twice daily to relax. If you are experiencing achiness, try to observe the anxious thoughts that accompany pain and let go of them.

Meditation can be combined with virtually any natural therapy.

MASSAGE (FOR BREAST LUMPS)

Because of its physiological and emotional benefits, massage can open the door to a whole new world of comfort and relaxation. Depending on what techniques are used, massage can help to transform you during periods of emotional stress, but can also invigorate you when you are feeling depleted. Specific techniques may be used for relieving a variety of conditions including breast discomfort.

Massage of the breast tissues can reduce some of the pain and swelling common during stages of fibrocystic breast disease. The massage warmup (in Chapter Three) will loosen tissue and promote relaxation. It can also promote a feeling of being centered and of emotional well-being during discomfort. Ask a helper to read the instructions and apply the techniques for you (see "Massage," Chapter Three). Then massage the breasts as described below.

Massage can be used in conjunction with any alternative therapy, and is often combined with acupressure, aromatherapy, and chiropractic.

Breast Massage

Use the tips of your fingers to press gently on the skin while rubbing small circles into the skin. Begin from outside the nipple area and work to the circumference of the breast, repeating this movement around the entire circumference. Now cup your whole hand over the breast and gently use your fingertips to knead the tissue in a large, circular motion. Repeat around the circumference of the breast. Repeat on other breast.

NUTRITIONAL THERAPY (FOR BREAST LUMPS)

Three primary factors that can be influenced by nutrition have been linked to occurrence of benign cysts—surges in the hormone estrogen, large amounts of caffeine-containing substances, and saturated fat in the diet.

Coffee, tea, and chocolate contain compounds called methylxanthines that have been linked to incidence of fibrocystic breast disease. One theory is that these substances inhibit chemicals that thwart cell division, making breast tissue overactive. When cells continue to divide, they accumulate in small lumps throughout the breast. Thus, it's important to eliminate caffeine-containing substances from the diet, which include, coffee, tea, chocolate, soft drinks, and many over-the-counter drugs, including many of those marketed for premenstrual relief.

The link with saturated fat may be partially explained by the hormones fed to meat and dairy animals and to poultry that may be ingested when we eat animal foods. Thus, cutting back on saturated fats, while possibly the key to relieving breast disease, offers many other health benefits as well. For more information, see "Nutritional Therapy," Chapter Seven.

Controlling the levels of estrogen that occur in the body is not completely possible. Still, there are several conditions that affect estrogen levels. Being overweight allows the body's adrenal glands to produce additional amounts of estrogen in body fat, which may contribute to many estrogen-promoted conditions including breast disease. Keeping the liver, which is responsible for breaking down estrogen in the body, working properly may help to reduce symptoms of breast disease. Adequate levels of B-complex vitamins are necessary for the breakdown of estrogen. A nutrient-deficient diet or excessive fat intake can also detract from the liver's ability to function properly. Reducing foods that promote estrogenlike effects, such as animal products—especially chicken—apples, cherries, olives, plums, peanuts, and soy products, can also be helpful. Liver-cleansing foods like beets, carrots, artichokes, lemons, parsnips, and dandelion greens can help release the toxins from the body and improve liver function. Avoiding meat, coffee, alcohol, sugar, and fatty foods can also help the liver.

Other nutrients that have been found to reduce incidence of breast disease include iodine, vitamin E, and vitamin A. Vitamin E normalizes the circulating hormones. Vitamin A is important for detoxification of the body, helping the liver do its work. In addition, when symptoms are exacerbated by premenstruation, magnesium and vitamin B_6 can play a key role in relieving breast discomfort. Be sure to get adequate amounts of foods containing these nutrients. For more information, see "Nutritional Therapy," Chapter Four.

Finally, incidence of breast disease has been linked with reduced colon function; that is, women with fewer than three bowel movements per week seem to be more susceptible to breast disease than women with at least one per day. Because estrogen can be reabsorbed from the bowel, more numerous bowel movements means that substances will not remain long enough for this to take place. Eating a vegetarian diet, which increases bowel movements, has been shown to minimize the reabsorption of estrogen. Eating nonfat yogurt of the type that contains *Lactobacillus acidophilus* cultures (some popular commercial brands contain them and are labeled as such) can also minimize estrogen reabsorption.

For a list of natural food sources that contain the above nutrients, see "Nutritional Therapy," Chapter Three.

CYSTITIS

Cystitis, or inflammation of the bladder, is thirty times more common among women than men. Recurring cystitis has become widespread, creating a great deal of frustration and discomfort for women. Cystitis usually occurs when bacteria from the bowel or vagina gets into the urethra, the tubelike vessel that channels urine from the bladder to be released from the body, and climbs up into the bladder. A woman is particularly vulnerable to bladder infection for several reasons. Because the female urethra is much shorter than the male urethra, it is much more accessible to invading organisms. In addition, because they are so close to the vagina, the urethra and bladder can become bruised or inflamed as a result of sexual intercourse. Intercourse may create pressure that blocks the usual signals for urination, thus allowing bacteria in the bladder to remain for longer periods of time and increasing possibilities for infection. In addition, pregnant women are at twice the risk for developing cystitis.

Once displaced bacteria enters the bladder, it begins to

act hostilely, provoking an immune-system attack. Depending on the other factors involved, the bacteria is either destroyed by the immune system, swept from the body through the urine, or develops into infection.

The most common type of bacterial infection, *E. coli,* is believed to have long, sticky fingers, or *pili,* which allow it to attach to most surfaces. The bladder's defense against such bacteria is found in its lining, which contains a substance called glycosaminoglycan that reduces bacterial adherence and infection. Its final defense against infection is urination, when the bladder washes bacteria from the body. So the longer the delay before urination, the more vulnerable one is to infection.

Most clinicians believe that the primary reason for delayed urination is simply habit. Thus, women who are prone to cystitis may be helping themselves a great deal by simply drinking more fluids to wash bacteria from the body and by urinating more frequently.

Some of the symptoms of cystitis include the urge to urinate frequently, burning upon urination, lower abdominal pain, and malodorous or dark urine. If cystitis is recurring, it will develop into a kidney infection about half of the time. Recurrent kidney infections can eventually result in permanent kidney damage.

When cystitis is recurrent, there are several factors believed to contribute. A sexual partner may carry the disease and may reinfect a woman after she has overcome the illness. Thus, the partner should also be treated for bacterial infection. Some women may have bladders that are particularly susceptible to bacterial infection because their cell linings are easy for bacteria to adhere to.

Allopathic treatment for cystitis usually involves antibiotics, which is the number one cause of vaginitis, another recurring infection among women. The cystitis-vaginitis cycle accounts for a large number of office visits. While serious infection should be treated allopathically to avoid any kidney complications, natural medicine offers a variety of alternatives for combating mild cystitis before it develops into a full-blown infection and for preventing recurrence.

ACUPRESSURE/ACUPUNCTURE (FOR CYSTITIS)

Energy balance in the body's meridians is essential for preserving health according to the ancient Eastern therapies of acupressure and acupuncture. However, bladder infection can arise when an imbalance leads to either an excess or deficient condition. For example, there can be an excess of heat and/or dampness in the bladder, an excess of cold, or a deficiency of yin, resulting in fire. Thus, both acupressure and acupuncture treatment entail resolving the imbalance that has led to this condition.

Described below are some acupressure remedies for bladder infection. Unless otherwise noted, you should press each acupressure point firmly but gently for two to three minutes, or until you feel relief. For further instructions on how to apply acupressure, see "Acupressure," Chapter Three. A visit to an acupuncturist would involve more in-depth treatment.

While acupressure is a gentle, safe treatment when used properly, some precautions should be taken. Acupressure should *not* replace standard medical care for serious infection. Consult a physician first.

- *Conception vessel 3:* Find this point about one fingerwidth above the pubic bone.

- *Conception vessel 2:* This point is situated on the upper border of the pubic bone, in line with the bellybutton.

- *Liver 3:* This point is located on the top of the foot in the depression beyond the juncture of the metatarsal bones of the big and second toes.

- *Liver 2:* You'll find this point on the top of the foot on the web between the first and second toes near to the margin of the web.

AROMATHERAPY (FOR CYSTITIS)

The strength of the essential oils found in plants combined with the powerful sense of smell form the basis for aromatherapy. A valuable tool during cystitis, aromatherapy can be used to relieve fluid retention, to promote relaxation, and restore the balance in mind and body. Described below are two suggested applications of aromatherapy: in a massage and in a bath. Unless otherwise noted, you should notice results right away, and do not need to continue therapy after your condition is improved. For a preventive treatment for maintaining balance and health, see "Aromatherapy," Chapter Three.

Precautions: Do not use aromatherapy as a *primary* treatment for cystitis.

To Relieve Fluid Retention

Massage.   The following massage will have an overall rejuvenating effect by relieving fluid retention in the body and thus promoting recovery as bacteria is washed from the bladder: Mix six drops each of parsley and pine oil in a carrier oil. Ask a friend to massage this into your abdomen and lower back according to these instructions:

First apply oil on the side you're working. To massage the lower back, begin at the lower curve of the spine and, using both thumbs side by side, apply pressure about a half-inch away from the spine, working down one side of it. Use a fast movement for a stimulating effect and a slow movement for relaxation. Finish at the coccyx (the "tail" of the spine), then begin again, working down the other side of the spine. Try to apply pressure at the same intervals on each side. Apply oil to the other side of the body. To massage the abdomen, use the palm of your hand to rub in a clockwise motion.

Bath. Use three drops each of juniper and lavender oils in a daily bath to soothe mind and body while the symptoms occur.

HERBS (FOR CYSTITIS)

Because herbs gently stimulate the body to heal, they provide a more favorable alternative than allopathic drugs for mild forms of bladder infection. Some effective herbs have been the favorite of women for treating cystitis and, when combined with nutritional therapies, can prevent recurrent cystitis.

Taking the herbs below in the recommended quantities may minimize some symptoms almost immediately, but benefits will increase incrementally over time. In all cases, do *not* take the herb for longer periods or in greater doses than recommended here.

Herbs should not be taken while using aromatherapy or homeopathy, but can be combined with most other natural therapies. For more information on herbs, see "Herbs," Chapter Three.

Uva Ursi (*Arctostaphylos uva-ursi*). Generations of families have used the leaves of this plant, a member of the same family as the rhododendron flower, as an antiseptic for healing urinary tract infections. Because of its diuretic qualities, this herb has gained favor among menstrual sufferers seeking relief from bloating and fluid retention. Uva ursi contains several chemicals credited with this effectiveness in the urinary tract. A substance called arbutin is chemically transformed in the urinary tract into an antiseptic chemical called hydroquinone. Diuretic chemicals, including ursolic acid, relieve fluid retention, while tannins are powerful astringents. A chemical called allantoin, used in wound healing and chapped-lip balm, is believed to promote the growth of healthy new cells. Together, these chemicals create a synergy that provides great relief from urinary symptoms. This herb can be useful for treating mild urinary discomfort, but for serious urinary problems like urinary tract infections, use the herb as a *supplement* to antibiotics. Although an effective diuretic, there is some evidence that uva ursi may stimulate uterine contractions. Therefore, it could possibly exacerbate menstrual cramps for some women.

Precautions: Because this herb may stimulate uterine contractions, it should *not* be used by pregnant women. Do not give this herb to children or elderly people. Do not use this herb as *primary* treatment for serious infections. Like all plant matter, tannins appear to have both carcinogenic and cancer-prevention qualities. While some experts believe that tannins may be particularly carcinogenic, others cite the need for better studies. Until more evidence is in, it is best to let caution prevail and to avoid herbs containing tannins if you have a personal or family history of cancer. A harmless side effect of this herb is its tendency to turn your urine a dark green or brown color.

Preparation: To minimize the unpleasant taste of this herb, soak it overnight in cold water. For an infusion, use two teaspoons of this herb per cup of boiling water for twenty minutes. Drink up to two cups per day. In a tincture, limit the dose to two teaspoons per day. Uva ursi tea is available commercially at your local health-food store. It is also commonly used in homeopathic formulas to treat gynecological problems.

Goldenseal (*Hydrastis canadensis*). The rhizome and roots of this member of the same family as the buttercup have long been treasured for their natural antibiotic effects. Goldenseal, called the "poor man's ginseng" has a variety of benefits, but its ability to heal infections caused by bacteria, fungus, and protozoa make it a valuable tool for healing cystitis and some types of vaginal infections. Goldenseal may also boost the production of the immune system to attack disease.

Precautions: Pregnant women should avoid this herb. It should not be given to children and elderly people.

Preparation: For a decoction, steep one and one-half teaspoons of dried root in one cup of water for twenty minutes. Drink no more than two cups per day.

NUTRITIONAL THERAPY
(FOR CYSTITIS)

Cranberries have long been the favorite remedy for relieving cystitis. While the popular belief is that cranberries acidify the urine to reduce infection, actually cranberries work by decreasing the invading bacteria's ability to adhere to the lining of the urethra and the bladder. Pure cranberry juice is recommended, especially since sugar is believed to have a detrimental effect on the body's healing abilities. However, commercial cranberry juice drinks, which contain only one-third juice, are more readily available. Drink one eight-ounce glass every hour for the first several hours, then do the same thing the following morning. If you are using pure juice, drink only three cups per day.

In general, a diet low in refined sugars and carbohydrates is recommended to maintain the internal environment of the body's organs, including the bladder. In addition, since many women with cystitis also develop vaginitis, following the dietary recommendations for vaginitis is also recommended.

Drink at least three liters of liquid each day to wash the bacteria from the body. The more fluid you send through the body's system, the more bacteria is taken with it from the bladder and urethra. Eating foods that are natural diuretics such as celery and strawberries can also help to wash away bacteria by promoting increased excretion of urine.

Garlic is wonderful for preventing and healing infections of all kinds. Thus, taking daily supplements of odorless garlic called Kyolic can be a useful tool for preventing or treating cystitis.

If you are taking antibiotics for cystitis, drinking buttermilk can be very helpful in preventing vaginitis, which often results from the imbalance of bacteria created inside the vagina. Once you stop taking the antibiotics, begin drinking buttermilk or taking supplements containing *Lactobacillus acidophilus* and other healthy bacteria twice each day, and continue for one week. (See Nutritional Therapy, Vaginitis, below).

ENDOMETRIOSIS

Endometriosis is a disease in which pieces of the endometrium spread inside the body and continue to act as if they were in the uterus by swelling, bleeding, and breaking up each month in conjunction with the menstrual cycle. Endometriosis most commonly affects the ovaries but can also affect the bowel or the lung and can spread to virtually anywhere in the body. About one in five women between the ages of twenty and thirty-five are believed to be affected by endometriosis, although some women may experience no symptoms and may be unaware that they have it. Endometriosis is a leading cause of painful menstrual cramps and accounts for half of all cases of infertility in women over the age of twenty-five.

Contrary to what many women may believe, endometriosis is not a precursor to cancer; in fact, less than 1 percent of women with endometriosis develop cancer, and seldom has the disease been shown to become malignant.

The most common theory of development of endometriosis is that some of the flow of menstruation is forced backward from the uterus through the fallopian tubes and showered upon the pelvic organs and pelvic linings. Tiny pieces of the endometrium then implant on organs and connective tissue and continue to respond to hormonal changes as if in the uterus—swelling each month with nutrients to support pregnancy, then shedding these nutrients during menstruation. Unlike the blood flow from the uterus, however, endometrial implants in the pelvic cavity lack a passage to leave the body. Thus blood flow is trapped and often inflames surrounding tissues, causing pain, irritation, and infertility. Endometrial complications can be exacerbated by the formation of scar tissue and adhesions, or dense, fibrous tissue, which becomes entangled with surrounding organs and interferes with their production. For example, infertility is often a result of implants that cloak the ovary and prevent ovulation. When left untreated, endometrial implants can spread to other organs as far as the brain.

Scientists are still unsure, however, why the disease develops in only some women, since retrograde, or backward, menstrual flow is believed to occur quite frequently. Hereditary factors are believed to contribute to the development of endometriosis as well—first-degree relatives of those with the disease are at greater risk for developing the disease.

While one in three women with endometriosis experiences no symptoms at all, half of all women experience pain. Symptoms are highly irregular and can vary from woman to woman and month to month. Nor do the symptoms offer any clues to the severity of the disease—a few tiny implants may cause excruciating pain in one person while widespread ectopic tissue may barely affect another. The most common symptoms of endometriosis are pain during menstruation and during intercourse and infertility, or the failure to ovulate. Endometriosis can affect even parts of the body distant from the uterus, so pain may radiate from locations, including from the pelvis to the rectum, leg, hip, lower back, shoulder, or head. Similarly, bleeding can emanate from a variety of sites, including the rectum, the bladder, or the lungs. If you have endometriosis, you may also experience symptoms such as nausea, vomiting, hypertension, fatigue, shortness of breath, tenderness around the kidneys, fever, urge for frequent urination, constipation, diarrhea, or spontaneous abortion.

Allopathic treatment for the disease can range from laser surgery to drugs and, commonly, hysterectomy, depending upon the severity of the disease. Next to uterine lumps (see below), endometriosis accounts for the most surgical procedures for gynecological problems in premenopausal women. Many allopathic surgeons are eager to eradicate the problem with a hysterectomy, but a woman may want to consider other options. Because she may believe that cancer is implicated, a woman may often feel obligated to have a hysterectomy, perhaps giving up her sense of femininity, pleasure, control over her own life and well-being. However, cancer is often not even a risk factor, and a women who learns to question her physician may learn that hysterectomy is only *one* of her options. Thus, she may decide to take a less invasive approach by using natural medicine.

With natural therapies, many women are able to manage or minimize the symptoms of disease or even prevent them in the first place. Natural remedies like herbs and nutritional therapy can work to lower levels of estrogen or progesterone that may contribute to the growth of endometriosis, and mind-body therapies like breathing and meditation can alleviate the physiological and emotional anxieties that likewise contribute to its development. In addition, relaxation techniques can help to minimize painful symptoms of the disease. In the case of any serious illness, alternative therapies should be undertaken only in consultation with your regular health provider, and should not substitute for your traditional medical care.

ACUPRESSURE/ACUPUNCTURE (FOR ENDOMETRIOSIS)

The Eastern therapies of acupressure and acupuncture, which maintain proper energy flow in the body's meridians to prevent illness, are very effective in treating endometriosis. In Chinese medicine, endometriosis can be caused by any of four patterns of disharmony that lead to blood stagnation: *chi* congestion, accumulation of cold, heat congestion, or *chi* and blood deficiency. Stagnant blood can be caused by stress and some oral contraceptives. It may also be caused by sexual intercourse during menstruation, which causes blood to flow backward in the uterus. It is important to remember that *chi* and blood keep each other in check just as yin and yang do; thus, stagnant blood can also be due to stagnant *chi*. The most frequent reason for *chi* congestion is stress. Because the liver is responsible for maintaining *chi* flow, *chi* congestion often causes liver stagnation. Other factors, such as surgery or trauma, eating too much food, dampness, or prolonged blood deficiency, can also lead to *chi* congestion.

Cold accumulation can also cause blood stagnation. This condition may result from excessive cold in the environment, or from overeating cold, raw, or damp foods that include sugar, oils, nuts, citrus fruits, and pork. If kidney yang, or kidney fire, decreases due to fatigue, sickness, or the use of recreational drugs, it may also lead to blood stagnation.

Heat congestion can cause blood stagnation as well, as a result of several factors. *Chi* congestion and liver stagnation with heat in the liver or gallbladder may be the cause, resulting in periods that are light, painful, and clotted, with some spotting in between periods. If the fire depletes the yin in the body, the fire is often prolonged. If this occurs, additional symptoms can include night sweats, hot flashes, and heat in the extremities and chest. Since the liver and stomach are closely related, if the liver gets heat, so does the stomach, which can then affect the intestines. In this case, a woman's period may be long, copious, painful, and clotted. This imbalance can also be worsened by eating fried or spicy foods and by drinking alcohol. Finally, an imbalance, with stagnant heat and blood, can consist of either hot energy above and cold below or hot inside and cold outside. An excess of stagnant blood but a deficiency of blood or *chi* or both may be present. This imbalance can cause symptoms of great menstrual pain, diarrhea, chills, and sometimes heaving.

The last type of endometriosis involves a deficiency of *chi*, which leads to a deficiency and stagnation of blood. Several factors can cause this energy imbalance, including exhaustion and eating nutrient-poor foods. The symptoms of this type of illness include a clotted menstrual discharge either early or late and light or extended menstrual flow. A woman may feel chilled, exhausted, and nauseous and have diarrhea.

Treatment by an acupuncturist will seek to correct these imbalances and is often very effective for controlling pain. In addition, women are generally instructed to avoid eating cold and raw foods, abstain from intercourse during menstruation, avoid dwelling on negative thoughts, and get enough rest, especially before and after menstruation. Acupressure points listed below may be helpful in relieving some of the symptoms of endometriosis.

For Severe Cramps

- *Spleen 8:* Locate this point about four finger-widths below the head of the tibia, in the depression on the inside border of the tibia.

For Heavy Bleeding

- *Spleen 1:* This point is situated where the nail of the big toe meets the skin, at the bottom inside corner. Besides pressing this point, a very effective way of reducing heavy flow is to hold an incense stick near the point until it is hot. Move the incense stick away briefly, then repeat again to reheat the point. Use this

method when you are already flowing heavily, not
before or after menstruation.

HATHA-YOGA (FOR ENDOMETRIOSIS)

See "Hatha-Yoga (for Breast/Uterine Lumps and Endometriosis)" presented earlier.

HERBS (FOR ENDOMETRIOSIS)

Herbs can be especially helpful for treating conditions
like endometriosis by providing several benefits. They can
promote liver functioning to assist in the breakdown of
estrogen in the body. They can also help to regulate estrogen or progesterone levels in the body, either of which
may contribute to endometriosis. Finally, many herbs can
relieve some of the symptoms of this disease, which can be
quite draining. Herbs gently soothe and restore our balance so that we can undertake the challenges that we face
on a day-to-day basis.

Taking the herbs below in the recommended quantities
may minimize some symptoms almost immediately, but
benefits will increase incrementally over time. In all cases,
do *not* take the herb for longer periods or in greater doses
than recommended.

Herbs should not be taken while using aromatherapy or
homeopathy, but can be combined with most other natural
therapies.

For more information on herbs, see "Herbs," Chapter
Three.

To Promote Liver Functioning

See "Herbs for Breast/Uterine Lumps and Endometriosis."

To Reduce Estrogen Levels

See "Herbs for Breast/Uterine Lumps and Endometriosis."

White Willow (*Salix alba*). The bark of this favorite herb has been popular since ancient times as a potent pain reliever. White willow may be most useful to women with endometriosis and fibroids because of its soothing properties as a pelvic sedative and an anti-inflammatory agent and its antispasmodic action.

Precautions: Do not give this herb to children or elderly people. Pregnant women should avoid it.

Preparation: For a decoction, steep two teaspoons of the dried root in one cup of boiled water for twenty minutes.

Vitex (*Vitex agnus-castus*). If your endometriosis is linked with elevated progesterone levels, this herb can be quite helpful because it supplies amounts of progesterone that are gentler than the body's own supply. The body takes in the herbal progesterone and releases the more potent form. It can also be helpful to women with endometriosis or fibroids because of its qualities as a pelvic sedative and antispasmodic agent.

Precautions: Pregnant women should avoid this herb. It should not be given to children and elderly people.

Preparation: For an infusion, steep one teaspoon of the dried herb in one cup of boiling water for fifteen minutes. Drink no more than three cups per day.

HYDROTHERAPY
(FOR ENDOMETRIOSIS)

Pain relief is one of the strengths of hydrotherapy, which combines the metabolic effects of water with the restorative properties of heat and cold. The application described below is useful in treating both endometriosis and uterine lumps. The sitz bath, which relieves pelvic pain, is one of the oldest hydrotherapy techniques known. Use the application for a sitz bath described in "Hydrotherapy," Chapter Four, but with some modifications. Use only the pelvic bath. Eliminate the footbath. And instead of drawing either a hot or cold sitz bath, alternate between them. Sit for three minutes in warm water, then thirty seconds in cold water. Do this three times. This technique will promote energy flow in the pelvic area. The hot water promotes blood flow, while the cold water causes a pumping action. Besides increasing energy flow, this technique also can promote release of endometrial tissue.

Another effective treatment for both endometriosis and uterine lumps are castor-oil packs placed over the uterus. Castor-oil packs improve circulation and provide soothing relief. For information on how to apply these packs, see "Hydrotherapy (for Osteoarthritis)," Chapter Nine.

Making a paste from bentonite clay and placing over the uterus can provide marvelous results for endometriosis and uterine lumps. Bentonite clay removes the toxins in the uterus, relieving sluggishness and having a restorative effect. Apply paste daily for three weeks of the month. Do not use during menses.

MEDITATION (FOR ENDOMETRIOSIS)

See "Meditation (for Breast/Uterine Lumps and Endometriosis)."

NUTRITIONAL THERAPY (FOR ENDOMETRIOSIS)

Because the same factors that promote endometriosis can also promote breast and uterine lumps, follow the dietary guidelines for promoting liver health and reducing estrogen levels in the section on "Nutritional Therapy (for Breast/Uterine Lumps and Endometriosis)." If anemia has become a problem, follow the dietary guidelines given in the section later in this chapter on "Uterine Lumps."

PSYCHOTHERAPY (FOR ENDOMETRIOSIS)

Women with uterine dysfunction such as endometriosis and uterine lumps may be suppressing feelings of anxiety related to sexual confusion, anger at a mate, or sexual abuse. Emotional and psychological factors can contribute to the development of these conditions because tensions become lodged in the reproductive organs and lead to physiological dysfunction.

Because you have suppressed such feelings many times, you may not be aware that they even exist. Often the problem stems from old hurts or concerns, perhaps even from childhood. Certainly issues of sexual abuse or assault can affect your sexual identity. But even factors that seem minor, like a disagreement with a mate, can actually have a deeper effect on your emotional life. Such physiological conditions may be related not only to sexuality, but to being a whole woman. You may have fears about your future, your job, or your mate, and you may be denying yourself the role of womanhood because of that fear. A good question to ask yourself is, what is this symptom preventing me from doing?

Thus, psychotherapy can help you to discover the root of your anxiety or frustration so that you can remove the fixation in the part of your body that is blocked. Your psychotherapist may use hypnosis to help you discover these feelings. Another technique involves self-affirmations of your self, womanhood, and natural body processes, which can reinforce your new way of thinking. For example, you can avow that you love being a woman and accept all your bodily functions as natural and normal.

Psychotherapy can be used with virtually any other alternative therapy and, when combined with mind-body therapies like biofeedback (Chapter Two); breathing for relaxation, hatha-yoga, and hypnosis (Chapter Eight); and meditation can produce powerful results. Besides promoting relaxation, the latter therapies can heighten personal insight.

UTERINE LUMPS

Despite their deceptive name, uterine fibroid lumps, sometimes called *fibroids,* do not arise out of fibrous tissue but rather the muscular layer of tissue called the myometrium that underlies the endometrial lining of the uterus. Fibroids may be found either on the inside or the outside of the uterus, or within the wall of the uterus. Those on the inside are the most problematic even if small; they can cause heavy bleeding and infertility. Like breast cysts, fibroid lumps are often stimulated by estrogen. They increase in size during estrogen therapy and during pregnancy. Most fibroid lumps are benign—they shrink or disappear following menopause. There is only a one chance in two hundred that a fibroid is cancerous.

Fibroids affect as many as one in four women over age thirty-five, but often many women are unaware of them because they cause no symptoms. Fibroids have a hereditary component, being nine times more common among black women than white women. Since lumps are believed to be stimulated by unopposed estrogen, birth control pills —which contain progesterone—are thought to slightly reduce risk of fibroids. Weighing more than 120 pounds slightly increases your risk, weighing 140 increases it, and so forth. Being overweight promotes additional levels of estrogen in the body since it can be synthesized in body fat.

Fibroids can cause many symptoms, including mild to large distension of the uterus, which is common even when there are no other symptoms. This can cause a woman with fibroids to look as if she is in an early stage of pregnancy. Because fibroids tend to take up a lot of space in the uterus and make it swell, the uterus can push against neighboring organs like the bladder and the bowel, causing symptoms such as a frequent urge to urinate.

While some women experience very little discomfort from fibroids, about one third experience heavy bleeding during periods or bleeding between periods for several reasons: Because fibroids enlarge the uterus, the endometrium expands to cover this enlarged surface area, and more blood is shed during menstruation. In addition, because large fibroids can place pressure on blood vessels in the uterus, they can alter blood flow. Finally, fibroids can stimulate areas of excess cell growth (hyperplasia), which are more responsive to hormones and tend to bleed more heavily. When heavy blood loss occurs from fibroids, many women become anemic.

Despite the fact that many women are able to live well with fibroids, almost one third of all hysterectomies are performed to remove them. Less common are myomectomies, or removal of only the lumps. But this surgery, besides inducing unnecessary trauma on the body, can present other problems as well. Removal of fibroid lumps is particularly likely to produce adhesions, or scar tissue that sticks to other surfaces. Adhesions can cause chronic pain or lead to infertility. While hysterectomies for fibroids are often unnecessary, the following are clear indications that hysterectomy is necessary: rapid growth of fibroid lumps, which could be a sign of cancer developing in the lump; uncontrolled bleeding; and excessively large tumors as they could interfere with the normal functioning of other nearby organs. However, even with very large fibroids— some women have reported them to weigh twenty pounds or more—many women experience no discomfort and no adverse symptoms. Even rapid growth of the fibroids is not a clear-cut sign that fibroids are cancerous—fibroids tend to grow in spurts, increasing rapidly for a while, then remaining dormant.

Natural medicine, however, offers nutritional and herbal therapies to minimize symptoms and sometimes to reduce the fibroids themselves.

HERBS (FOR UTERINE LUMPS)

Herbs can provide several benefits for women with uterine lumps. They can promote liver functioning to assist in the breakdown of estrogen in the body, which may contribute to the development or progression of fibroids. Herbs can also help to regulate estrogen levels in the body, which may contribute to this condition. Finally, many herbs can relieve some of the discomfort caused by this disease, which can be quite draining.

Taking the herbs below in the recommended quantities may minimize some symptoms almost immediately, but benefits will increase incrementally over time. In all cases, do *not* take the herb for longer periods or in greater doses than recommended below.

Herbs should not be taken while using aromatherapy or homeopathy, but can be combined with most other natural therapies. You should consult with your health-care provider before undertaking any herbal therapy.

For more information on herbs, see "Herbs," Chapter Three.

To Promote Liver Functioning

See "Herbs (for Breast/Uterine Lumps and Endometriosis)."

To Reduce Estrogen Levels

See "Herbs (for Breast/Uterine Lumps and Endometriosis)."

Goldenseal (*Hydrastis canadensis*). The rhizome and roots of this member of the same family as the buttercup have long been treasured for their natural antibiotic effects. But many women with uterine conditions from endometriosis to uterine lumps are finding goldenseal valuable in calming the uterus and reducing heavy blood flow. For more information, see "Herbs (for Cystitis)," presented earlier.

Nettles (*Urtica dioica*).   The leaves and stems of this old-time favorite have been popular since ancient times to reduce inflammation of the joints during arthritis and gout. But those with uterine lumps may benefit also from its ability to soothe the uterus as well by relieve pain.

Preparation: For an infusion, steep one teaspoon of dried herb in a cup of boiling water for fifteen minutes. Drink no more than four cups per day. For a tincture, take one teaspoon once each day.

Precautions: Do not give this herb to children or elderly people. Pregnant woman should avoid taking this herb because it may stimulate uterine contractions. Be careful to avoid touching the stinging, hairlike bristles found on this plant. Large doses of nettles may cause stomach upset.

Wild Yam (*Dioscorea villosa*).   The roots and the rhizome of this popular herb have traditionally been used to prevent miscarriages, but women with inflammatory problems have long valued its soothing relief for a variety of gynecological conditions from breast and uterine lumps to endometriosis. Wild yam is effective because it helps to balance the female hormones in the body. But its effects are many—wild yam is an antispasmodic, an inflammation-fighter and a diuretic. It may also be helpful in relieving morning sickness during pregnancy.

Preparation: For a decoction, steep one and one-half teaspoons of the herb in one cup of water for twenty minutes. Drink no more than three cups per day.

Precautions: Pregnant women should avoid taking more than one cup per day of this herb. It should not be given to elderly people and children.

HYDROTHERAPY
(FOR UTERINE LUMPS)

See "Hydrotherapy (for Endometriosis)."

MEDITATION (FOR UTERINE LUMPS)

See "Meditation (for Breast/Uterine Lumps and Endometriosis)."

NUTRITIONAL THERAPY
(FOR UTERINE LUMPS)

Women who experience heavy bleeding from fibroids
may experience anemia. Although clinicians don't agree as
to what constitutes anemia and when it should be treated,
there is no question that if you are looking pale and experience symptoms of heart palpitations, dizziness, fatigue, or
shortness of breath (especially if, for example, you are not
exerting yourself and your environment is comfortable),
you may be anemic and should consult your physician.
Fortunately, treatment for anemia is not extensive or complicated. It simply means you must eat foods that are rich
in iron and possibly take iron supplements.

Studies have shown that increasing iron-rich foods and/
or taking iron supplements can not only reduce anemia but
also can decrease bleeding from fibroid lumps! Iron supplements are recommended if you are unable to consume
enough iron-rich foods or if anemia is severe. Most people
have difficulty in absorbing iron from traditional supplements, however, so taking bioactive supplements such as
spirulina may be helpful (see Nutritional Therapy, Chapter
Four). If bioactive supplements are not available in your

area, traditional supplements can be useful, especially if combined with iron-rich foods. However, avoid synthetic iron supplements called ferrous sulphate. Organic iron called hydrolyzed-protein chelate works well.

If your anemia is not severe—that is, you occasionally experience shortness of breath and feel tired—you can probably improve your condition to some extent just by eating a meal full of iron-rich food sources. Red meat has one of the highest concentrations of iron from animal sources—next to liver, which is also full of toxins—so if you are not a vegetarian, one way to boost iron levels initially may be to eat a roast beef sandwich or piece of steak. In addition, iron-rich foods from animal sources or foods that contain vitamin C, if eaten simultaneously with iron from plant sources, increase the body's absorption of the latter. So you might augment the steak with a baked potato. If you include a tablespoon of blackstrap molasses, which contains almost one third of the recommended daily allowance (RDA) of iron, you will boost iron levels even further. Regularly eating red meat can lead to other health problems and is not recommended, so once you bring iron levels up to normal, establish a well-balanced diet that contains a variety of iron-rich foods.

If you are a vegetarian, you can boost iron levels by combining iron-rich plant foods with iron supplements. Bioactive supplements such as spirulina are a terrific source of natural iron. Good plant sources of iron include mustard greens, potatoes, pumpkin seeds, and fortified breads.

If you take supplements, be sure not to overload on them—perhaps taking only two to three times the RDA—because ingesting too much iron has been linked with heart problems. In addition, excessive amounts of iron can lead to a deficiency in calcium, a vital nutrient for women. Don't be surprised if your urine turns a tinge of green if you're taking supplements—that's the result of iron that the body cannot absorb being excreted.

Some foods, like tea and the bran found in whole grains, decrease iron absorption by the body and should be avoided in large amounts during anemia. Adding milk to tea can reduce the adverse effect. Similarly, vitamin B_{12}, necessary for the production of red blood cells by the liver, is often deficient in a strict vegetarian diet. Thus, eating foods that are rich in vitamin B_{12} is another way of counteracting anemia.

Some studies have shown that a deficiency in vitamin A can lead to heavy bleeding as well. Symptoms of vitamin A deficiency include black rings around the eyes, dry hair, nail shadowing, dry cervix, and furred tongue.

In addition, because high levels of the hormone estrogen are believed to contribute to the development and growth of fibroid lumps, minimizing levels whenever possible is recommended. See "Nutritional Therapy (for Breast Lumps)."

For a list of natural food rich in these nutrients, see "Nutritional Therapy," Chapter Three.

Psychotherapy (for Uterine Lumps)

See "Psychotherapy (for Endometriosis)."

VAGINITIS

Because of its recurring nature, vaginitis is said to account for almost 10 percent of all visits to the gynecologist. Thus, women who suffer from vaginitis have a lot to gain from natural medicine, which offers a variety of therapies to relieve minor infections and prevent its recurrence. Vaginitis can be any of several infections of the vagina that lead to symptoms of inflammation, itching, or burning, a smelly, heavy, or discolored discharge; and frequent and/or painful urination.

Vaginitis can develop a number of ways. The most common cause is the use of antibiotics to treat cystitis, or bladder infection. Normally an acidic chemical balance is maintained in the vagina by *Lactobacillus* bacteria so that fungi can not proliferate. When an environmental factor alters this balance, such as antibiotics that kill the beneficial *Lactobacillus*, the vagina becomes vulnerable to overgrowth of fungus, and infection often develops. Other causes of vaginitis include sexual transmission; decreased levels of estrogen, such as after menopause; depressed immunity as a result of serious illnesses; poor nutrition; pregnancy, or certain drugs, like steroids.

The most common type of vaginitis is called *Candida albicans,* sometimes called *Monilia,* a yeastlike fungus that normally inhabits the bowel and may also get into the vagina. *Candida albicans* can also be a systemic disease that causes symptoms throughout the body, the nutritional treatment for which is the same as for vaginal *Monilia. Candida* overgrowth can be promoted by the use of the birth control pill, wearing synthetic underwear or nylons that prevent moisture from evaporating, as well as the factors listed above. If a condom is not used during intercourse, a sexual partner can carry *Candida* and cause reinfection. Diet can also play a major part in the development of *Candida.* A diet high in refined sugar and carbohydrates, both of which become glycogen after being processed, lowers the acidic content of the vagina and can allow the fungus to grow.

If you have a serious infection, you should see an allopathic physician immediately to obtain a diagnosis. In addition to causing discomfort and pain, full-scale vaginitis can also be a sign of another condition that has developed, such as a sexually transmitted disease or inflammation of the cervix. Allopathic treatment for vaginitis usually involves antifungal creams that do not get at the cause of the condition that leads to such a high rate of recurrence or, worse, antibiotics that are suspected to cause birth defects and genetic mutations. Thus, intervening with natural therapies when the infection first takes hold—for example, when you experience the slight urge to urinate frequently and there is a slightly abnormal discharge—is recommended.

Some caution should be used in diagnosing your own condition, however. Many vaginal infections won't hurt, itch, or emit an unpleasant smell. Consequently, in order to identify infection, you must first be able to recognize changes in your vaginal secretions. Healthy secretions won't irritate your vagina, they will only feel wet. Variations in secretions during the menstrual cycle are normal. Although discharges may change in consistency, they will usually remain transparent or milky white in color. During ovulation, however, vaginal discharge will usually become stretchy, watery, clear, and profuse, while after ovulation and following menstruation, secretions will become sticky and opaque. During pregnancy, vaginal secretions will increase. Normal secretions may have a mild odor.

If you have *Candida* vaginitis, the most prominent symptom is itchiness of the vulva, but it may accompany sensations of burning, and/or swelling of the vagina or vulva. In fact, painful urination is more frequently a sign of vaginitis than it is of cystitis. In addition, vaginal secretions may become thick, curdy, and white, sometimes with a strong yeastlike smell. If you have trichomonas vaginitis, caused by a protozoon transmitted through sexual intercourse, vaginal discharge can be a frothy greenish-yellow with a foul smell and cause burning and itching. Atrophic vaginitis, caused by waning estrogen levels during menopause or following oophorectomy (removal of the ovaries), often produces a thin, watery discharge with itching or burning. Gardnerella vaginitis, caused by overgrowth of anaerobic bacteria, results in a grayish and sometimes frothy discharge, often without other signs of vaginitis.

Natural therapies have a lot to offer women who suffer from vaginitis. You can curb the development and progression of vaginitis through herbal preparations, acupuncture, and nutritional therapies.

ACUPRESSURE/ACUPUNCTURE (FOR VAGINITIS)

Maintaining proper energy flow is the key to alleviating imbalance and, thus, illness, according to the philosophy of the ancient Eastern therapies of acupressure and acupuncture. However, most infections, including vaginitis, can result when an energy imbalance leads to a number of conditions. For example, vaginitis may result from an external invasion of cold, deficiency of *chi* and/or blood, dampness and heat in the "lower burner," the lower part of the uterus, deficiency of the spleen or stagnation of liver *chi*. Acupressure treatment can relieve mild vaginal symptoms of itchiness, while an acupuncturist can diagnose the pattern of imbalance and then provide treatment to restore it.

Described below are some acupressure remedies for relieving vaginitis. Unless otherwise noted, you should press each acupressure point firmly but gently for two to three minutes, or until you feel relief.

• *Heart 8:* When a fist is made, this point is located where the tip of the smallest finger rests, between the fourth and fifth metatarsal bones.

- *Conception vessel 3:* Find this point about one thumb-width above the top of pubic bone, in line with the bellybutton.

- *Conception vessel 2:* This point is situated on the upper border of the pubic bone, in line with the bellybutton.

Acupressure should *not* replace standard medical care for serious infection. For further instructions on how to apply acupressure and additional precautions, see "Acupressure," Chapter Three. A visit to an acupuncturist would involve more in-depth treatment.

HERBS (FOR VAGINITIS)

Natural herbs can provide a good alternative to allopathic treatment for vaginitis. Herbs stimulate gentle and unique effects that are not found in drugs. Some herbs have an antibiotic quality for treating certain types of vaginal infections. Other herbs that produce estrogenlike effects may be useful for relieving vaginitis due to vaginal atrophy during menopause. When combined with other natural therapies, healing herbs can be very effective in alleviating recurrent vaginitis.

Taking the herbs below in the recommended quantities may minimize some symptoms almost immediately, but benefits will increase incrementally over time. In all cases, do *not* take the herb for longer periods or in greater doses than recommended below. You should consult with your health-care provider before undertaking any herbal therapy.

Herbs should not be taken while using aromatherapy or

homeopathy, but can be combined with most other natural therapies.

For more information on herbs, see "Herbs," Chapter Three.

Goldenseal (*Hydrastis canadensis*). The rhizome and roots of this member of the same family as the buttercup have long been treasured for their natural antibiotic effects. Goldenseal has the ability to heal infections caused by bacteria, fungus, and protozoa, making it a valuable tool for healing most types of vaginitis. For more information, see "Herbs (for Cystitis)."

Nettles (*Urtica dioica*). The leaves and stems of this old-time favorite have been popular since ancient times to reduce inflammation of the joints during arthritis and gout. But vaginal sufferers favor it for its success in fighting infections. Nettles also have a diuretic effect, making them effective in counteracting high blood pressure and a variety of other ailments. For more information, see "Herbs (for Uterine Lumps)."

Licorice (*Glycyrrhiza glabra*). The roots and rhizome of this member of the bean family have been shown effective in treating a variety of infections, but are especially helpful in fighting the fungus responsible for vaginal yeast infections.

Precautions: Pregnant women should avoid this herb. It should not be given to children and elderly people.

Preparation: For a decoction, steep one teaspoon of dried root in one cup of boiling water for twenty minutes. Drink no more than two cups per day.

NUTRITIONAL THERAPY
(FOR VAGINITIS)

Dietary factors play a big role in the health of the vagina, and consequently there are many dietary tools that can help to keep vaginitis under control and prevent its recurrence. In general, a diet low in refined sugar and carbohydrates and fats will help to maintain the natural balance in the vagina and prevent infections of all types.

In addition, there are a number of dietary factors that have been linked with *Candida albicans*, the most common type of vaginal infection. Eating a pint of nonfat yogurt three times each day can be helpful in relieving mild infection because it contains active cultures of *Lactobacillus acidophilus*, a type of "good" bacteria found in the reproductive and gastrointestinal tract that is responsible for fighting infection and maintaining a healthy reproductive system. Many commercial brands may contain these cultures, but purchasing brands that are labeled as such is the safest approach. Capsules of *Lactobacillus acidophilus* may also be inserted directly into the vagina twice each day until symptoms begin to disappear and then once a week as a preventive measure if you are prone to developing vaginitis. Also, several companies now sell supplements that incorporate *Lactobacillus acidophilus* in the same proportions found in the body, preventing the possibility of imbalance. Available in a liquid or a powder form that can be mixed with water, the solution can be taken orally or used as a vaginal douche.

Another way to balance the natural flora in your body is to eat an avocado with a vinaigrette dressing of two parts olive oil and one part organic cider or wine vinegar every day for two weeks. A diet of sunflower seeds and whole grains will help build and maintain resistance against fungal infections.

Avoid foods that contain refined sugar and carbohydrates, both of which are notorious for altering vaginal balance. Some nutritionists even recommend eliminating fruit from the diet until infection is eliminated because it contains natural sugar. Many nutritional experts also believe that infection can be worsened by eating foods containing yeast, like breads, and other molds, like cheese, because they increase mucus levels in the body. Thus, eliminating breads, cheese and alcoholic drinks (which also contain yeast) can be helpful in maintaining the health of the vagina. Other foods linked with *Candida* that may be avoided include MSG, vinegar, milk (contains sugar), coffee and tea (because they increase urinary excretion of sugar), smoked meats, fish, and sausages.

Certain nutrients are also believed to promote vaginal health, and ensuring adequate amounts of them in the diet may be helpful in preventing and treating vaginitis. Vitamin C restores acidity to the vagina and promotes immune-system functioning. Both vitamins A and E can reduce vaginal inflammation and infections and promote immune-system functioning. Vitamin A is also necessary for the maintenance of healthy tissues in the vagina. A long-term deficiency of vitamin B_{12} has been linked with vaginitis, so eating foods high in this nutrient, a difficult task for strict vegetarians, is needed. Taking a B-complex vitamin pill may be in order, which also may be useful in counteracting vaginitis that occurs as a result of vaginal atrophy during menopause. If you feel you must take supplements of any of these nutrients, avoid yeast-based vitamins. Bioactive supplements provide an excellent natural source of B-complex vitamins.

Garlic has wonderful preventative and healing benefits for women with vaginitis. When taken orally, it can kill *Candida*, but don't use it as a suppository—it will sting like mad. Taking daily supplements of odorless garlic, called Kyolic, can be a useful tool for preventing vaginitis.

If you are taking antibiotics for cystitis, drinking buttermilk, which contains *Lactobacillus* bacteria, can be very helpful in preventing vaginitis. As soon as you stop the antibiotics, begin drinking buttermilk or taking supplements containing *Lactobacillus acidophilus* and other healthy bacteria (see above) twice each day, and continue for one week.

CHAPTER SIX

Pregnancy

Few processes of the human experience seem as miraculous as pregnancy, in which the body is able to orchestrate a complex metamorphosis for nurturing a new life.

One of the first signs of pregnancy is delayed menstruation, which can be a result of other factors as well (see Chapter Four). If accompanied by breast changes, including swelling and darkening of the nipple, delayed menstruation is usually a positive indication of pregnancy. If you suspect you are pregnant, be sure to have a pregnancy test performed. If your test results are positive, your delivery date will be calculated from your last menstrual cycle, not the suspected date of conception, for a total period of forty weeks.

Over the next nine months, your body will undergo great hormonal changes to provide for the developing baby. The body doubles or triples its levels of some hormones, and secretes two additional hormones full-time, progesterone and human chorionic gonadotropin (HCG). The uterus will change dramatically, enlarging rapidly from the size of a pear in the first month to about seven or eight times its size at delivery. Your bones and ligaments will loosen so that the pelvic region can widen enough for a successful delivery.

The body undergoes dramatic metabolic changes as well. It produces more protein in all of its tissues, increases levels of fats and cholesterol in the blood, and extracts additional levels of calcium, phosphorous, potassium, iron, and other nutrients from foods for the growing infant. These changes begin gradually in the first month when the embryo is in its early stages. By the end of the first month of pregnancy, the embryo does not look quite like a human because it has a "tail" formed by its spinal cord. The head and neck make up most of the embryo, and the heart is beating and circulating blood. By the second month, the backbone, spinal canal, limbs, and organs are formed, and the muscles and bone are developing. The appearance of a "tail" in the undeveloped embryo disappears now. Perhaps most exciting, the development of the sexual organs in the third month allows clinicians to determine with specialized testing whether the fetus is a boy or a girl. With the embryo's liver and kidney developed, these organs can perform their unique functions. By now, the developing infant begins to move by contracting its muscles rapidly and continuously, although you won't be able to detect movement for another month. Fetal movement is usually an indication of its healthy status, but if you don't feel constant movement, don't be alarmed—the embryo moves quite frequently without being detected. The fetus breathes with oxygen supplied by the placenta, an organ that develops in the third month to support and protect it —not the gaseous oxygen we breathe as adults, but a liquid called surfactant, which is pumped into the lungs.

And while the growing baby thrives from the enormous metabolic transformations taking place in the body, the mother-to-be becomes quite exhausted, especially during the first eight to ten weeks. Besides fatigue, an array of other side effects are common during the first trimester. Once the uterus begins to expand, it increases pressure on the bladder, making the mother-to-be feel the urge to urinate frequently throughout pregnancy. Increased activity in the reproductive tract also can result in bladder infection (cystitis) or vaginal infection (vaginitis). Treating the latter infection with medication may harm the fetus, but natural therapies provide a safe and effective therapy. (For more information, see Chapter Five).

Levels of the HCG hormone, which cause the common complaint of nausea or vomiting called "morning sickness" that can usually occur in the evening or any time of the day, are produced in the first trimester. As early as the second month of pregnancy, the breasts are stimulated by levels of the hormone prolactin, which prepares for breastfeeding and may cause breasts to become tender, hard, lumpy, or leaky. Elevated hormone levels can cause a variety of other effects as well. They can alter the appearance of the skin by heightening pigmentation and moles and by producing red spots or weblike stains. Hormones can also cause or intensify sensitivity to the sun, so fair-skinned women who are prone to sunburn should avoid excessive exposure. Women who tan well, however, may luxuriate in the additional glow of the sun's rays. Because hormones stimulate the mucous membranes in the nose and head, sinus headaches may begin now and continue throughout pregnancy. With the hormones altering the entire chemical composition of the body, a woman may feel upset, irritable, or even turbulent. However, as the body begins to adjust to the enormous changes of the first trimester, fatigue diminishes, breast tenderness and nausea disappear, and most other complaints become minimal, leading to lifted spirits in the second trimester.

Now is when most women experience the "glow" of pregnancy, the surge of euphoria felt especially by first-time mothers. Now is also when a woman's body shows the first sign of pregnancy caused by a rise in amniotic fluid, sometimes very suddenly, in the fourth month. Others become aware that you are expecting, sometimes heightening the excitement of pregnancy. Women who have had several children may "show" much earlier than others because the inner wall of the abdomen is more relaxed and gives way more easily. Now is also the time when uterine contractions begin and continue throughout the rest of the pregnancy. Fetal development, of course, continues at a rapid rate.

In the fourth month, the rapid heartbeat of the fetus—which is sometimes twice that of an adult—can be detected. And for the first time, a woman can actually feel the developing baby move—at first feeling more like gas and later becoming unmistakable. Pregnancy may feel more "real" now! By the fifth month, the fetus is about ten inches long and weighs barely a half-pound. The skin and the facial features are fully developed and appear wrinkled, a condition that will disappear when fat covers the body. A cheesy-looking substance covers and protects the whole body, including the face. During examinations, or perhaps at home, some of the growing infant's anatomy can be felt through the skin. By the sixth month, the fetus's skin, a bright and shiny red, is covered by lanugo, a fine hair.

During the final trimester of pregnancy, additional weight gain leads to a series of other discomforts that compound the frustration of being unable to move gracefully, and many women feel as if they have entered a three-month marathon. Most women gain between thirteen and thirty-five pounds during pregnancy. The average gain is 24.5 pounds—2.5 pounds the first trimester, 10.8 pounds the second trimester and 11.2 pounds the third trimester. About three pounds of weight is fluid retention, mostly in the face and fingers, due to increased circulatory needs of the fetus—the mother's body provides vital nutrients to the fetus and carry its waste away. Constipation often results from hormonal changes that relax the colon, coupled with increased pressure on the bowel. While not every woman experiences them, "stretch marks," dense white or brown lines, sometimes cover bulging areas of the skin, usually around the breast, buttocks, and abdomen. Stretch marks usually become thin and white and barely distinguishable some months after delivery.

Other hormonal changes affect the skin. Dark patches of brownish color sometimes appear on the face, but disappear some months after delivery. Muscle cramps, especially in the legs, are usually related to a calcium shortage (see "Nutritional Therapy"). Women also experience swelling of the legs and ankles, although it is not caused by fluid retention but by increased pressure of the uterus on the veins of the legs. Uterine pressure can also cause varicose veins, swelling of the veins in the legs and ankles, and hemorrhoids, because extra weight bears down on the veins of the anus. Unless swelling is accompanied by high blood pressure, headaches, and/or visual disturbances, it is not a sign of toxemia, a rare but serious complication of pregnancy.

The extra uterine weight also affects a number of other body functions. Less space in the lung area means less room for expansion and, coupled with the increased demand for oxygen during pregnancy, may make pregnant women feel short of breath. Some women may experience dizziness during this period due to low blood pressure caused by uterine pressure on the major blood vessels of the body. Uterine weight also causes a women to compensate by leaning backward—hence the common picture of the swaggering woman in her final month of pregnancy— causing backache.

Not surprisingly, all of these discomforts can make sleeping difficult; this, coupled with the fatigue women often experience during the third trimester, give the latter stage of pregnancy its reputation for being quite taxing on body and mind. Despite the desire for relief from the many ailments of this stage, it's important for women to avoid taking aspirin during the third trimester, when it is likely to affect the unborn child and/or cause complications during delivery.

During the third trimester, the developing baby begins the final stage of growth. By about seven months, the fetus's development is almost complete, and its chances of surviving on its own increase incrementally with each day. The eyes that were fused shut are now open, and the neonate begins to grow hair. The developing baby now weighs about six to seven pounds and is about eighteen to twenty inches long. Almost ready for its debut in the world, the infant grows stronger until, finally, somewhere near the fortieth week of pregnancy, a timer goes off and the uterus begins to contract. The cervix, the small opening to the uterus, begins to grow thinner and wider—labor has begun. Minutes or hours later, when the infant is finally pushed from the body, the lungs begin to breathe in oxygen and the fluid surfactant simultaneously stops flowing. The end of a nine-month journey and the beginning of a new one as a thriving human being occurs with the sound of the baby's wail. To the proud parents, this is the first day of a long future together as a new family.

While every parent wants to give birth to a healthy infant, such accomplishments do not happen without effort. A mother-to-be must be careful to nurture the growing infant not just after birth, but *before* birth as well. Because a woman is often unaware that she is pregnant for several weeks after the fetus has substantially developed, she should maintain a healthy lifestyle at all times. Most important is to avoid exposing the fetus to environmental and health risks that may have adverse effects during various stages of its development, effects that may not be evident until later in life.

A pregnant woman should eat a balanced diet, avoid alcohol, drugs, and cigarettes, and minimize work-related hazards. Eating a balanced diet is important to avoid causing deformities and other ailments in the newborn. Malnutrition is also the leading cause of premature birth. Health conditions related to body size can contribute to difficulties for both mother and infant—women who are obese are more likely to experience hypertension, have prolonged or difficult labor, or suffer from gestational diabetes during pregnancy. In addition, they may give birth to larger babies. Conversely, women who are underweight or gain less than average weight during pregnancy generally give birth to babies who are underweight.

Tobacco is another factor that affects the developing infant, sometimes leading to lower birthweight or even premature delivery. Drinking alcohol should be avoided during pregnancy—even as few as two to four drinks per week—because it doubles the risk of spontaneous abortion. Heavy drinking can cause even more harmful results —retarded growth and brain and spinal abnormalities, a condition called fetal alcohol syndrome. Recreational drugs like cocaine can lead to hyperactive and jittery habits in the infant; and heroin can lead to an addicted baby. When the mother has a sexually transmitted disease like herpes or syphilis, it can result in miscarriage, birth defects, or even death of the child.

The working woman must also consider on-the-job hazards that can affect the developing baby. Women whose jobs involve heavy physical activity, long hours, or high stress should try to ease up on these conditions during pregnancy because they can have harmful effects on the developing infant. Exposure to certain chemicals and gases should be avoided. Some special precautions should be taken by an X-ray technician, for example, to avoid exposure to radiation. Similarly, an operating room professional should minimize exposure to anesthetic gases; an employee of a paint, glass, ceramic, or battery manufacturing plant to heavy metals; and a laboratory or dental employee to mercury vapors.

Women who give birth later in life are often concerned about possible complications of birth. However, birth defects are not as prevalent as commonly believed. Only Down syndrome, a birth defect in which inherited genes cause some physical and mental abnormalities, is age-related. The risk for Down syndrome does not become significant until women reach their forties, and can be diagnosed early in pregnancy with a procedure called amniocentesis.

By affording you the opportunity to become more involved in prenatal care, natural medicine can greatly heighten the sense of pleasure you derive from nurturing a new life. Natural therapies offer a pregnant woman a way to minimize many health risks, provide holistic prenatal care, and greatly improve her comfort level during pregnancy. Because success rates vary with different therapies listed below, experimenting will be helpful. Be sure to perform therapies according to your own abilities and comfort. Most important, do not use natural therapies as a substitute for prenatal care from a certified nurse-midwife or licensed physician.

ACUPRESSURE/ACUPUNCTURE

The energy-based Eastern therapies of acupressure and acupuncture can help to alleviate many discomforts associated with pregnancy by stimulating proper energy flow in the body. Discomfort can result when any of the body's meridians become stuck, blocked, or reversed, often upsetting the energy pattern in other parts of the body as well. Acupressure and acupuncture treatment involve a variety of techniques for redirecting energy flow.

Described below are various acupressure remedies for common complaints during pregnancy. Unless otherwise noted, you should press each acupressure point firmly for two to three minutes, or until you feel relief. For further instructions on how to apply acupressure, see "Acupressure," Chapter Three.

While acupressure is a gentle, safe treatment when used properly, some precautions should be taken. You should never use acupressure to treat any other ailments, or press any other points during pregnancy except those listed below. There are a number of points forbidden during pregnancy, and some acupuncturists may want to wait until the second trimester to treat a pregnant client, feeling that the energy of the fetus needs to be firmly established before redirecting energy; however, acupuncture treatment is safe and effective for treating complaints throughout pregnancy, including morning sickness, abdominal pain, edema, vaginal spotting, low back pain, and frequent urination. Be sure to tell anyone doing body work on you that you are pregnant! (For more information, see "Acupuncture," Chapter Three.) Acupressure or acupuncture should *not* replace standard prenatal care by a licensed physician or certified nurse-midwife.

For Relieving Morning Sickness (Cramps, Nausea, Vomiting)

- *Pericardium 5:* You can find this point on either forearm, four finger-widths above the center of the inner wrist crease between the tendons.

- *Pericardium 6:* You can locate this point about three finger-widths from the upper crease of the wrist on the inner forearm between the two tendons.

- *Stomach 36:* This point is located on the calf, four finger-widths below the bottom of the kneecap, one finger-width outside the shinbone. The point is on a muscle, which you can feel move if you flex your foot.

For Breast Discomfort

- *Conception vessel 17:* This point is situated on the center of the sternum (breastbone), level with the fourth intercostal space.

- *Stomach 18:* You'll find this point in the fifth intercostal space, one rib below the nipple.

- *Stomach 34:* This point is located about two inches above the outer, upper border of the kneecap.

- *Pericardium 6:* You can locate this point about three finger-widths from the upper crease of the wrist on the inner forearm between the two tendons.

For Heartburn and Indigestion

- *Stomach 43:* You can find this point on the top of the foot in the hollow between the second and third toes where the two bones meet.

For Hemorrhoids

- *Governing vessel 20:* This point is situated in the center of the top of the head in line with ears.

- *Bladder* 57: Locate this point directly below the body of the calf muscle.

AROMATHERAPY

Aromatherapists utilize the powerful sense of smell coupled with the effectiveness of essential oils found in plants to stimulate a variety of health benefits. The physiological and emotional effects of aromatherapy can activate mind and body to heal a range of conditions during pregnancy from morning sickness to poor circulation.

Listed below are suggested remedies for common complaints related to pregnancy. Unless otherwise noted, you should notice results right away, and do not need to continue therapy after your condition is improved. Once balance and health are restored, however, you may want to incorporate a preventive treatment into your daily routine for keeping the body and spirit well (see "Aromatherapy," Chapter Three).

Precautions: You should avoid the following essential oils, which promote the onset of menstruation, during the first two trimesters of pregnancy: clary sage, rosemary, and melissa.

To Improve Circulation

Massage. Massage the legs with an oil consisting of a base of two ounces soy oil and three drops of wheat-germ oil, plus two drops each of rose, lemon, and cypress oils. Apply oil to the legs, and, beginning with the feet and working up to the thighs, squeeze gently with the fingers. Apply pressure with the thumb to the inside of each ankle, about one thumb-width from the backbone, and to the back and center of each thigh. Both improve circulation. The ankle pressure will also help to relieve fluid retention.

For Hemorrhoids

Massage. Mix three drops of geranium oil to one ounce of vegetable oil and massage into rectal area whenever symptoms occur.

For Nausea

Massage. Prepare a mixture of four drops of rose oil to two teaspoons of vegetable oil and massage into the solar plexus when symptoms occur.

For Constipation

See "Aromatherapy," Chapter Four.

For Insomnia

See "Aromatherapy," Chapter Four.

For Emotional Upset

See "Aromatherapy," Chapter Three.

BREATHING FOR RELAXATION

During pregnancy, the body's need for oxygen increases dramatically because of the additional work done for the fetus. Thus, in order to accommodate the increased needs, a pregnant woman needs to breathe more deeply. Women

who breathe in substantial amounts of oxygen can also reduce fatigue and increase nutrient delivery to cells of the
developing infant. Women who are relaxed also enhance
their ability to promote an easier labor and delivery. In
addition, by inducing relaxation, women can minimize the
discomforts associated with pregnancy. Healthy breathing
has another benefit as well. It can prevent the body's stress
response to anxiety-provoking circumstances, which increases susceptibility to stress-related conditions and illnesses. Rapid, shallow breathing is the first indication of
the body's stress response and, consequently, the most efficient way to avert it. Try the belly-breathing practice in
"Breathing for Relaxation," Chapter Three.

EXERCISE

While exercise during pregnancy was once discouraged,
it is now known to have many benefits. Exercise improves
circulation, increases energy levels, and can counteract hypertension and gestational diabetes, both of which increase
the risk of premature birth. In addition, aerobic exercise
supplies a natural form of pain relief for the discomforts
associated with pregnancy. Of course, during pregnancy,
activity that is too strenuous can have harmful effects, and,
if you've never exercised before, pregnancy is not the time
to undertake a rigorous exercise program. In addition, no
matter how much you exercised before pregnancy, exercise physiologists recommend that you cut back dramatically by the sixth month. For all pregnant women, however, gentle exercise can provide wonderful physiological
and emotional benefits, from enhancing delivery to minimizing cramps and muscle tension.

During pregnancy, exercise improves circulation, which
can minimize swelling in the legs and feet and alleviate leg

cramps. Exercise can also fight fatigue by increasing energy levels and alleviating insomnia. Exercise is known to increase fetal movement, which promotes health of the growing baby. Studies also show that women with gestational diabetes who perform moderate exercise of even the upper arms can lower blood sugar and reduce the symptoms of diabetes.

But keeping exercise at a moderate level during pregnancy is necessary for several reasons. During pregnancy, the body's cardiovascular and respiratory systems are taxed with the additional needs to supply the fetus. Metabolism is affected. Most of the body's fat and carbohydrates, normally burned in exercise, are salvaged for the augmented nutritional needs of the developing fetus. Instead, the body burns its blood sugar during exercise, which is why moderate exercise is so beneficial for women with gestational diabetes. But too much exercise can tax oxygen requirements and deprive the growing baby. Too much exercise can also raise the temperature in the placenta surrounding the fetus, which cannot cool itself.

Thus, exercise physiologists recommend that pregnant women exercise between three and five times per week for fifteen to twenty minutes, not including a warmup and cool-down period, which should be included in each exercise session. However, excessive stretching should be avoided to avoid damage of ligaments, already loosened by hormones to facilitate delivery. Exercising less frequently or only intermittently can actually stress the body, so be sure to maintain a regular program. Be sure to drink plenty of water before and during exercise to prevent dehydration.

Swimming or light jogging are safe and easy exercises for the first five months of pregnancy, while walking can be performed throughout the entire pregnancy. Even walking at a leisurely pace of three miles per hour, five times per week, provides wonderful health benefits. This routine lowers cardiovascular risk by raising the "good" HDL cholesterol and provides psychological benefits. Aerobic exercise like jogging also causes the body to release its natural pain-killing endorphins and enkephalins. To learn how to establish a walking regimen, see "Aerobic Exercise" in Chapter Three.

In addition to these exercises, the preventive exercises listed below can help to keep you in shape during pregnancy and to prepare for delivery.

Precautions: You should not begin or continue an exercise program except under the supervision of a licensed physician or certified nurse-midwife. If you have any specific medical conditions like placenta previa or an incompetent (expanded) cervix, exercise should be avoided. If you have health risks like obesity, being underweight, or if you have juvenile diabetes, exercise should be avoided except under the approval of your caregiver. Because of risk associated with extreme heat, avoid exercising on particularly hot or humid days or when you have a fever. Also, do *not* use a sauna or hot tub during pregnancy.

During First Trimester

Now is the time to get in shape for the months ahead when your physical stamina will be challenged. By performing these exercises to tone and strengthen muscles of the abdomen, you are preparing your body to support the weight gain of future months. Strong abdominal muscles can alleviate backache, a common complaint during the second and third trimester of pregnancy, when the mother-to-be compensates for extra weight in the abdomen by leaning backward.

See the *yoga situp, abdominal rock,* and *single-leg lift* exercises in "Hatha-Yoga," Chapter Seven.

During Second Trimester

Now that you are carrying additional weight you should be careful to avoid leaning too far back and thereby stressing the spine, which can cause backache. Keeping the abdominal muscles in good working order can also prevent backaches in these and future months. Leg exercises can help to prevent cramps by increasing the circulation in the legs. Exercise can allow you to thrive at this unique time in your life!

Modified Leg Lifts. Lie on your left side. Bend your left elbow, and bring your hand under your head to gently support your upper body. Bend your left knee about forty-five degrees, and lift your right leg slowly and gently into the air with the right knee bent. Raise it as high as is comfortable or about one and one-half feet to a count of four. Lower your right leg to a count of four. Perform six to ten leg lifts. Repeat this exercise while lying on the right side of the body. The object of this exercise is to increase circulation in your leg and gently strengthen the muscle to increase your comfort level, not to build large muscle tissue, so don't be concerned about your pace or the number of repetitions—perform this exercise according to your own abilities.

Good-Posture Promoter. With knees slightly bent, stand against a wall so that your shoulders and buttocks are touching the wall. To a count of five, gently push your lower back toward the wall until it touches or as close as you can comfortably go. Hold for a count of ten. Repeat the exercise six times.

Advanced Abdominal Exercise. If you have practiced the abdominal exercises listed above during the first trimester, you will most likely be able to perform this exercise, which requires good abdominal strength. Sit down with your knees bent and about one and one-half feet from the floor and your feet flat on the floor. Place your arms criss-cross on your chest and lean back several inches to a count of four or as far as you can go without losing your balance. Bring your upper body back to the original position to a count of four. Perform this exercise six to ten times or as long as is comfortable.

During Third Trimester

In the third trimester, extra weight decreases mobility, which can result in fatigue. Thus, exercise is helpful in improving overall circulation and promoting higher energy levels. In addition, exercises that stretch the muscles used during childbirth can ensure a smoother delivery. Any exercise during the third trimester should be performed while standing or sitting halfway upright. Lying flat on your back should be avoided because the uterus puts pressure on the main vein leading to the heart and slows blood flow, lowering blood pressure.

Delivery Enhancer. Sit on the floor with knees bent and the soles of feet together (or as close as you can bring them). Clasp your hands around your ankles, and use each elbow to push gently down on the knee. This stretches the muscles around the groin. Do this six to ten times. As you become more flexible, your knees will go farther and farther to the floor.

Upper-Body Stretch. Stand with back straight, knees bent and legs apart about one and one-half feet. Put your hands on your hips. Without losing your balance, slowly bend forward from the waist to a count of four. Resume your original position to a count of four. Now repeat, but this time swing your upper body to the right to a count of four. Bring back to the center to a count of four, then to the erect position to a count of four. Now lean forward again to a count of four, this time swinging to the left to a count of four. Next, swing to the center to a count of four, then to the right to a count of four. Swing back to center to a count of four, then back to the upright position. Repeat this exercise three to four times or as long as you feel comfortable.

Sitting Upper-Body Stretch.   Sit on the floor with legs crossed in front of you or as close to this position as possible. Gently twist your torso, neck, and head as far to the right as possible to a count of four. Put your right hand on the floor for support, and hold for a count of four. Gently swing back to the center position to a count of four. Repeat for the left side. Repeat the entire exercise three to four times or as long as you feel comfortable.

HOMEOPATHY

Homeopathy is a perfectly safe and effective medical system during this important time in a woman's life. It provides an array of treatments for relieving symptoms that are common throughout pregnancy, from first-trimester morning sickness to third-trimester backache. Healing actions don't overpower the body's own defenses, an important consideration during pregnancy; instead, remedies gently activate the body's inherent healing powers using substances that would produce a similar set of symptoms if given to a group of healthy individuals over a period of time. In fact, homeopathic healing will not be stimulated unless the remedy symptoms correspond quite well with individual symptoms. Conversely, if the wrong remedy is taken, no harmful effects will result; the treatment will simply have no effect.

If you are treating yourself, it's important to match your feelings and physical symptoms as closely as possible with the remedies listed below, just as a homeopath would. Unless otherwise noted, take a dose of 6c no more than twice daily for a maximum of seven days. Stop taking medication once symptoms begin to disappear. If your medication has no effect, it usually indicates that you have taken the wrong remedy. In that case, review your symptoms and, being as specific as possible, match them to another remedy. Also, you should always consult your doctor or certified nurse-midwife before taking any remedy while pregnant.

Homeopathy may be used in conjunction with some therapies like acupuncture and hypnosis (Chapter Eight), or psychotherapy (Chapter Two), but it should generally not be used simultaneously with aromatherapy or herbs because the former's essential oils may inactivate the homeopathic solution, as will coffee, alcohol, tobacco, perfumed cosmetics, and pungent household cleansers.

For Back Problems

- *Kali carbonicum:* If your back feels strained, your muscles fatigued, and dragging pains in the lower and middle back are nagging you, this remedy may be very helpful.

- *Arnica:* If your back feels quite strained due to overexertion and poor posture because of the extra weight you are carrying, try this for relief.

For Breast Discomfort

- *Conium maculatum:* If your breasts feel slightly tender because of swelling, taking this can provide a great benefit.

- *Bryonia:* If tension and stiffness in the breasts are making you feel very uncomfortable, this remedy may give you great relief.

- *Belladonna:* This remedy can be very helpful if your breasts are tense and stiff, with red weblike stains or lines across them.

For Cramps in Calves

- *Nux vomica:* If your legs and the soles of your feet are cramping and feel better when you rest, and your arms and hands feel numb and without circulation, and your conditions worsen in the cold, this can bring you real relief.

- *Veratrum viride:* Try this if you feel a tension in the calves that feels better when you walk or apply heat.

For Constipation

- *Bryonia:* If you feel uncomfortable during movement, your stools are very hard and dry-looking, and you are often very thirsty, this can provide you with great benefit.

- *Sepia:* If congestion in the lower gastrointestinal tract causes you to feel pain, and your stools are large and very solid, taking this remedy may bring you relief.

- *Sulphur:* Try this for relief if your rectum is inflamed, or you have hemorrhoids and your stools are hard and irregularly shaped.

For Heartburn and Indigestion

- *Sulphur:* You may reap great benefit from this if heartburn is worse late in the morning, you have a poor appetite except a craving for sweet foods, and you are constantly thirsty.
- *Colchicum:* If just the sight of food makes you nauseous, and your stomach feels like it is cold inside, this may help.

For Hemorrhoids

- *Pulsatilla:* If you feel great pain during bowel movement, this could help you.
- *Nux vomica:* If hemorrhoids constantly ache but are worse after drinking alcohol or coffee, and you are constipated, this remedy could benefit you even if not pregnant.

For Morning Sickness

- *Pulsatilla:* If nausea is worse in the evening, this may help you a great deal.
- *Nux vomica:* Try this for relief if nausea is worse upon waking and you vomit even small amounts of food.
- *Ferrum:* If you vomit after eating and feel nauseous intermittently throughout the day, you may gain benefit from this remedy.

For Shortness of Breath

- *Aconite:* If your heart beats rapidly, you feel as if you can't get enough air, and you constantly feel faint, all of which makes you feel anxious and scared, this may help you.
- *Ipecac:* This may help you if you constantly feel nauseous and as if you can't get enough air, and you sometimes faint.

For Insomnia

See "Homeopathy," Chapter Seven.

For Emotional Symptoms

See "Homeopathy," Chapter Seven.

IMAGERY

During pregnancy, a mother-to-be may spend a great deal of time celebrating the imminent joys ahead, but the expectations of motherhood can weigh heavily on her as well. A woman may worry about her transition from career woman to mother or whether she still possesses the vigor to nurture an infant, for example. Or she may be concerned that she is not yet ready for the responsibilities of motherhood. Imagery can be helpful in counteracting these negative images so that a woman doesn't fall victim to a self-fulfilling prophecy, where one's fears are actualized, often because they are given so much attention. These fears are, after all, only imagined and not probable or sometimes even possible! If you envision yourself coping well in the role of motherhood, you can promote the actualization of a positive course of events. Relaxation imagery can be useful to relieve emotional and physiologic stress that can have harmful effects on the body. Relaxation imagery can also be helpful in relieving some of the discomforts associated with pregnancy, which can become intensified by feelings of anxiety. Try the relaxation imagery technique (see "Imagery," Chapter Three) twice daily to relax. If you are experiencing discomfort and fatigue, try to incorporate some invigorating images into your exercise. Using vivid and meaningful images will enhance the benefits of this therapy.

Imagery can be used in conjunction with any natural therapy, but offers its greatest advantages when combined with biofeedback (Chapter Two), hypnosis (Chapter Eight), and other relaxation techniques.

MASSAGE

Natural massage therapy can provide just the right amount of relaxation and soothing relief that is needed during pregnancy. When the discomforts of swelling contribute to fatigue, leaving you feeling emotionally and physically drained, a massage can restore your feelings of wellness and joy. Quick strokes can invigorate the body and mind and give back a feeling of being centered on the most trying days, while slower strokes can soothe and relax. While massage should not be performed in the pelvic area during pregnancy, it can relieve poor circulation in the body, especially in the legs, caused by increased uterine pressure on the veins. Massage can restore circulation in the legs and feet, and relieve the emotional tension that may accompany discomfort.

The massage warmup can be helpful in the first five

months of pregnancy, but be sure to avoid massaging the pelvic area. In later months, the technique described below can be helpful in relieving leg cramps and aches. Ask a helper to read the instructions and apply the technique for you. (For more information about massage and related precautions, see "Massage," Chapter Three.)

Massage can be used in conjunction with any alternative therapy, and is often combined with acupressure and aromatherapy.

To Relieve Swelling and/or Muscle Spasms in Legs and Ankles

Lie on your side or on your back with your upper body supported by several pillows so that you are leaning at least at a forty-five-degree angle from the bed or couch. Ask your helper to apply oil using long, gliding strokes to the top of the legs, beginning with the feet and working up to the thighs. Now begin with the feet by applying pressure with the thumb to the inside back of the ankle. This should improve circulation and help to relieve fluid retention. Rub the sole of the foot from heel to toe with a gliding motion to improve circulation. Gently pull on each toe. Now begin with the feet again, and squeeze the skin gently with the fingers until you reach the thighs. You're ready to release tension from the deep muscles. Start with the calves, taking large amounts of skin and muscle into your hands and working the tissue by squeezing, kneading, and rolling. Work your way up the thighs. You'll feel the tension roll from the muscles as the tissue softens. Finish by lightly brushing the entire area with your fingertips.

MEDITATION

While expecting, a pregnant woman may expend excessive energies thinking about her new lifestyle and role as a new mother, how the father will adapt, and any number of other concerns. Thus, meditation is a great therapy for quieting the mind and soothing the spirit so that calmness once again can reign. Meditation is simple yet effective and can be accomplished in as little as fifteen minutes each day. It involves a state of mindful awareness in which thoughts are not competing for attention—in fact, they are only distractions from the peaceful state of inactivity integral to meditation. Meditation is particularly beneficial during the gestational months because it promotes not only physiological relaxation, but mental release as well, replenishing body and mind. Relaxation can not only have benefits during labor and delivery, but can help to quell the discomforts during pregnancy that become intensified by anxiety. Try the practice meditation (see "Meditation," Chapter Three) twice daily to relax.

NUTRITIONAL THERAPY

All of an unborn's nutrients come from the mother. Yet caloric intake should increase only slightly during pregnancy. The body adapts to pregnancy by squeezing out additional nutritive value from foods. In general, pregnant women who perform moderate amounts of exercise should consume only an extra 300 calories each day. Very athletic women should consume another 200–300 calories per day, for a total of 500–600 extra calories per day.

The need for most nutrients also increases slightly, however, so it is most important during pregnancy to avoid "empty-calorie" foods, or those that are calorie-dense but nutrient-poor. Eating foods that are loaded with valuable nutrients or even taking a daily multivitamin pill and mineral supplement is recommended if you are unable to consistently consume sufficient amounts of these foods. However, taking large doses of any vitamin or mineral is unnecessary and can even have a detrimental effect on the developing infant. Large doses of vitamins A, D, and K, for example, have been shown to be harmful to the fetus.

The body's need for protein increases slightly during pregnancy, from about 45 grams per day to 60 grams per day, so women should consume an additional serving of protein-rich food per day. Vitamin C demands also increase slightly from 60 to 70 milligrams per day, the total amount for which can be found in a large orange.

Metabolic functions related to the growing fetus also increase the body's need for B-complex vitamins. Vitamin B_6 is needed to metabolize proteins and fat, for a total requirement of 2.2 milligrams per day. Vitamin B_6 with nutritional yeast has been also shown to be an effective deterrent of nausea symptoms. Three B-complex vitamins necessary for the fetus's metabolic functions—niacin, riboflavin, and thiamine—increase slightly to 17 milligrams, 1.6 milligrams, and 1.5 milligrams, respectively.

To accommodate the body's blood supply to the growing infant, several nutrients also need to be augmented during pregnancy. Vitamin B_{12}, necessary for production of red blood cells and the absorption of iron, increases to 2.2 milligrams. To shuttle oxygen around in the red blood cells, iron is needed in double the amount. Inadequate levels of iron can cause the heart to work much harder to pump oxygen and lead to great fatigue or even risk for cardiac disease. Eating iron-rich foods with orange or other citrus juice can enhance iron absorption, while milk and milk products inhibit its absorption. While it may take some extra effort to double consumption of iron-rich foods, it is certainly possible. Certain foods interfere with iron absorption, however, namely, tea, bran of grains, and oxalic acid found in, ironically, spinach, which contains high levels of—alas—unavailable iron. Because of this mineral's poor absorption by body, allopathic medicine traditionally offers pregnant women iron supplements of between 400 and 900 milligrams per day! But excessive levels of iron have been linked with heart disease, although conflicting studies exist. In addition, iron supplements increase the need for oxygen, pantothenic acid, and other nutrients, as well as inhibit absorption of vitamins E, A, and C, all of which are essential during pregnancy. For more information on increasing iron levels, see "Nutritional Therapy (for Uterine Lumps)," Chapter Five.

Another B-complex vitamin, folic acid, is vital for the formation of genetic materials and red blood cells. One study showed that taking supplements of folic acid in the first trimester of pregnancy was effective in lowering incidence of spina bifida, a malformation of the spinal cord. Ensuring an adequate daily total of 400 micrograms—an increase from 180 micrograms—of folic acid–rich foods can minimize such occurrences and promote better health.

Requirements for iodine increase slightly from 150 to 175 micrograms, levels of which are easily obtainable in iodized salt and other food sources like sea vegetables. Too little iodine has been linked to cretinism, a condition of impaired physical movement and mental ability, and too much iodine has been linked with mental retardation, so, again, balance in the diet is necessary.

A woman's demand for zinc, essential for cell growth, increases by 3 milligrams for a total of 15 milligrams during pregnancy. Excessive levels of zinc have been linked to premature birth and birth deformities, while a deficiency of this mineral has been associated with nervous-system dysfunction, and underweight newborns. While the requirement for copper remains the same, a deficiency in copper has been associated with premature birth.

Of course, a woman's body must also supply enough nutrients for the development of the fetus's skeletal system. Thus, the need for the macrominerals calcium and phosphorus increase from 800 to 1,200 milligrams, while the need for magnesium increases by 40 milligrams to 320 milligrams during pregnancy. Vitamin D, necessary for calcium synthesis by the body, doubles, for a total of 10 micrograms needed in the diet. Despite all the hype, milk is not the best source of calcium because it can inhibit this mineral's absorption as well as iron absorption. Nonfat yogurt and dark, leafy green vegetables are much better sources of calcium. For more information on increasing calcium levels in the body, see "Nutritional Therapy (for Osteoporosis)," Chapter Nine.

Besides eating a balanced diet, pregnant women should also avoid some foods that can have detrimental effects on the growing fetus. Caffeine use has been linked with birth abnormalities, miscarriage, and premature birth. Besides being found in coffee, tea, chocolate, and soda, caffeine can also be found in some medications, including common pain relievers. Be sure to check the label. In addition, the tannins in tea can inhibit absorption of iron, levels of which are essential during pregnancy. Avoid alcohol; in moderate amounts it has been linked with miscarriage; in great amounts with fetal alcohol syndrome.

Diuretics should also be avoided. Not only do they lower the body's supply of potassium, an important mineral for the growing fetus, but they also minimize the fluid in the body that is necessary to circulate additional nutrients and carry wastes from the fetus.

During pregnancy, you may experience several conditions resulting from hormonal or other changes in the body that may be relieved with nutritional therapy. They include:

Nausea

Nausea, which is caused by increased levels of hormones during the first trimester, can be minimized by eating small amounts of food all day to keep food in the stomach. Drinking peppermint tea and eating crackers, which soak up hydrochloric acid in the stomach, should be helpful. Even moving slowly and calmly can help to alleviate nausea because mild anxiety tends to aggravate it.

Heartburn

In the latter months of pregnancy, heartburn is often caused by the uterus pressing on the abdomen, pushing food up the esophagus. Sitting upright while eating small amounts of food may help to relieve this condition.

Constipation

Constipation, caused by the relaxation of the colon and increased pressure of the uterus on the bowel, can be relieved by eating foods that are high in fiber such as whole grains, fresh fruits, and vegetables. Drinking plenty of liquids, especially cold water, can help to restore movement in the bowel.

Leg Cramps

Early-morning leg cramps that develop during pregnancy are not a sign of muscle strain as you might expect. Actually, they represent a calcium deficiency in the body, usually caused by the body's inability to absorb enough calcium. Drinking cow's milk, which contains substances that block calcium absorption, is a primary cause of leg cramps. Thus, pregnant women should obtain much-needed calcium from nonfat yogurt and other natural food sources instead of milk.

For a list of natural foods containing these nutrients, see "Nutritional Therapy," Chapter Three.

CHAPTER SEVEN

Menopause

In the autumn of her life, a woman experiences a metamorphosis, a decade of dramatic physical, emotional, and physiological changes of a magnitude that surpass any other that she has experienced. When she completes this passage, she will have arrived at menopause, a new stage of her life. With the reproductive years concluded, she is free to pursue passions and goals. She may reevaluate her career and decide to move in a new direction. Emotionally, she can be more self-confident and speak her mind without fear of backlash. Without the concerns related to childbearing, she may experience a new sexual freedom. She is zesty, spirited, and adventurous, and yet she is wiser and more mature than before—she has the best of both worlds. In some cultures, she becomes matriarch and mentor, in others, she takes on a new position in society. In all cultures, she has a new place in the world.

But menopause was looked upon quite differently by American society in the late 1800s. It was once believed that women who were too learned, who used birth control, or enjoyed sex too much, and those who were insufficiently devoted to their family experienced the worst bouts with menopause, a disease that could cause everything from diabetes to diarrhea. Standard treatment for such a disease, besides reform and remorse, was no less than leeching or oophorectomy (surgical removal of the ovaries).

Today, menopause is recognized by the allopathic community as having a biochemical basis. However, allopathic medicine offers little to women except hormonal replacement therapy, a treatment with often thunderous side effects. Such a treatment may remedy the physiological symptoms of menopause, but makes irrelevant the psychological, emotional, and spiritual experiences of this passage. Natural therapies, in contrast, do not disregard the backdrop and setting of your life—factors like stress, community, exercise, nutrition—which shape your experience of health and illness. Natural therapies offer a variety of techniques for enhancing your comfort during menopause. Healing herbs, aromatherapy, and homeopathy can manage the hormonal changes within the body, while hydrotherapy and massage can soothe your ills and help to restore your body to a regular sleep cycle, commonly interrupted during menopause. Exercise and nutritional therapies are tools for curbing the bone loss that can occur beginning in the middle years, while yoga exercises can gently reduce aging effects in your body. Together, these therapies can aid in a smooth transition into the autumn of your life.

Before we look at specific therapeutic applications, let's first look at what occurs during perimenopause, the transitional five to seven years before ovulation ceases, and what happens following menopause. The reproductive years begin when a woman reaches menarche, a time in which she carries some 75,000 follicles, or premature egg cells. These eggs will be released from her ovaries for possible fertilization over the next three decades. Every month, the body stimulates secretion of a follicle-stimulating hormone (FSH), which promotes the development of a few of these follicles. As the follicles begin to mature, the hormone estrogen is secreted by the ovaries to promote changes in the reproductive organs. It causes the uterine lining, called the endometrium, to thicken with nutrients and blood vessels in preparation for a possible pregnancy. With these changes underway, a substance called leutinizing hormone (LH) is secreted, which causes the matured egg to be released from the ovary. This event, called ovulation, prompts the levels of FSH and LH in the body to drop and large amounts of the hormone progesterone (which means "for pregnancy") to be secreted. Progesterone promotes further buildup of the endometrium. If fertilization of the egg does not occur now, levels of estrogen and progesterone begin to drop dramatically. Within several days, menstruation will occur, which will prompt levels of FSH to be secreted and the cycle to begin again.

As we age, a transformation occurs. The ovaries begin to slow down and become less sensitive to chemical changes, and their supply of eggs begin to dwindle. The body stimulates secretion of greater and greater amounts of FSH and LH to promote follicle development. Despite increases by as much as fifteen times of FSH, chemical resistance is so great that the body often fails. In addition, the ovaries, with their egg supplies almost depleted, begin to slow down estrogen production. Instead of gradually tapering production, however, the ovaries sputter and reel, and estrogen levels dip and soar. In the latter stage of perimenopause, ovulation occurs only sporadically. Without ovulation, not enough of the hormone progesterone is released to cause changes leading to menstruation. Thus, irregular menstrual cycles and heavy periods are commonly experienced during perimenopause. Heavy periods result when buildup of the endometrium is not released until after ovulation—possibly two to three months or longer because of the less efficient system. A menstrual period that is three months late may be three times as copious. An erratic menstrual pattern can continue for several months or several years. Not until menstruation has ceased for one year can it be assumed that ovulation has stopped permanently. Heavy periods can also be a warning sign that another condition has developed, however. (See Chapter Five and Chapter Eight.)

The perimenopausal transition usually begins in the early to mid-forties. Because estrogen function affects so many other processes in the body, the dramatic dips and peaks of the hormone that occur during perimenopause unfortunately may result in a two- to three-year roller-coaster ride for many women. Fundamental body functions from sleep to eating to sex, as well as feelings of well-being, may be thrown off-kilter during this transition. Not surprisingly, psychological symptoms like irritability, fatigue, anxiety, insomnia, and depression are often the result. Other changes occur, too. Without a constant estrogen supply, the skin and hair may become thinner and drier. The vaginal walls begin to thin out and are drier and more prone to irritation. And surges in estrogen may cause cysts in the breasts. Together, this torrent of physiological and emotional change can greatly affect the quality of life for women during perimenopause. Happily, most of these disturbances disappear after menopause when estrogen production, although very minimal, at least becomes steady. For the first several years, however, when balancing mind and body is imperative, natural therapies can be very helpful for restoring harmony.

Perhaps the most upsetting symptom of menopause is the physiological phenomenon shared by about 75 percent of women: the hot flash. A hot flash may be a brief feeling of warmth in the face or upper part of the body, or it may be a dousing sweat followed by chills. Hot flashes are caused by hormonal fluctuations. They may last for a few seconds or a few minutes and may occur once a week or every hour. Some women experience them primarily during the day, others at night. When they occur at night, they often interrupt the sleep cycle. Interrupted sleep thwarts the body's ability to regulate its body temperature, thus exacerbating the cycle. During a hot flash, the blood vessels in the skin become dilated, and perspiration results. Surprisingly, the body temperature falls. Hot flashes vary from woman to woman and day to day. Feelings of anxiety and tension may precede the flash by seconds and may be accompanied by such physical sensations as dizziness, nausea, tingling in the fingers, or heart palpitations.

Because hot flashes are believed to be linked with estrogen levels, several factors can affect their severity. Generally, thin women, women who experience severe menstrual discomfort, and those with surgical menopause experience more intense hot flashes than others. Thin women have less body fat, where estrogen is primarily produced by the adrenal glands after menopause. Reduced stores of fat also deter such production during perimenopause, when estrogen peaks and ebbs, thus increasing hot flashes. Women who experience severe menstrual symptoms are believed to be very sensitive to hormonal fluctuations and so may also experience a more difficult transition during perimenopause. Also, women who have had an oophorectomy experience an abrupt drop in estrogen levels, resulting in more severe hot flashes than those felt by most perimenopausal women. Hot flashes, like most fluctuations that occur during perimenopause, will cease within a year or two. By menopause, the body is once again in harmony with the mind.

Predicting when menopause will occur is difficult. Half of all women stop ovulating before age fifty and half later than that. Factors like reproductive history and onset of menarche have little effect on menopausal onset; it seems to be largely a genetic attribute. Some factors do appear to influence onset a bit, though. Women who weigh more than 130 pounds tend to experience the change of life later than those who weigh less because larger amounts of estrogen can be made in the body fat. Women who experience menopause after age fifty are at double the risk of developing endometrial cancer and, after age fifty-five, are at double the risk of developing breast cancer. Menopause can develop prematurely, or before age thirty-five. Oophorectomy, of course, causes immediate menopause, but other factors can accelerate the process as well, including mumps, autoimmune diseases, and radiation therapy for treating cancer. Smoking hastens the onset of menopause because it causes the ovaries to cut back on estrogen production.

By the time menopause occurs, most of the fluctuations and emotional seesaw has ceased. The body's sex hormonal composition has changed entirely. While a small amount of estrogen is secreted in body fat by the adrenal glands, the levels of male sex hormone, testosterone, secreted in the body in small quantities prior to menopause, increase slightly. Many women experience an increased sex drive during this time, believed by some to be a result of this testosterone increase. Other women experience a lack of interest in sex, perhaps due to the vaginal dryness that accompanies menopause.

Other changes occur following menopause. The vagina begins to lose its tone and shape over the years if muscles aren't toned. Keeping sexually active is the best remedy for keeping the vagina lubricated and healthy. Skin and hair can also become a little drier at this stage. And, without estrogen, women go through accelerated bone loss for seven to ten years following menopause. Then bone loss stabilizes. This bone loss can be attributed to the cutback in estrogen, which plays a vital role in the body's calcium uptake, as well as in inhibiting loss of bone mass. Osteoporosis, a silent disease, can also begin accelerating when estrogen declines. However, its symptoms are not visible until it becomes the major cause of bone fractures in post-menopausal women. Some women are more vulnerable to bone loss than others (for more information, see Chapter Nine).

Some health risks increase for postmenopausal women. A woman's risk of heart disease increases to equal that of a man for several reasons. Levels increase of LDL cholesterol, the "bad" cholesterol that sticks to the arteries, and decrease of HDL cholesterol, the "good" cholesterol that sweeps LDL cholesterol from the arteries. Without estrogen, the blood vessels lose the elasticity that was important during the reproductive years, when pregnancy could dramatically expand a women's blood volume. And the body's metabolism slows, increasing the possibility of weight gain. Weighing more than 130 percent of your recommended body weight is an increased risk for heart disease.

Thus, taking care of yourself during the postmenopausal years is more important than ever before. Natural therapies are valuable in this regard; they're gentle and safe and can be practiced in your own home. Your transition to menopause is likely affected by a combination of lifestyle factors, thus, treatment with many therapies can enhance your comfort level.

ACUPRESSURE/ACUPUNCTURE

In Chinese medicine, menopause results when kidney yin, the water that sustains and cools the body, diminishes. Since yin influences the whole body, its decline can produce symptoms such as hot flashes, jittery feelings, and perspiration. A decrease in kidney yin can lead to several other reactions in the body. If kidney yin decreases, heart and liver yin can also decline, and yang, the fire of the body, can become more potent. An overbalance of yang, the energy of which naturally rises to the head, can result in hypertension and hot flashes. If an excess of yang influences the orb of the heart, it can result in the inability to sleep, oversensitivity, and even minor heart trouble.

The natural aging process can lead to other energy imbalances as well. When weakened kidney yin is accompanied by decline in kidney yang, the result can be feelings of depression and exhaustion as well as constant urination. When *chi* in the conception vessel becomes feeble, it may lead to moderate but continuous bleeding from the uterus, copious or irregular menstrual flow, and stomachache.

After assessing the energetic basis of your menopausal symptoms, an acupuncturist will choose the appropriate points to nourish the kidney yin and/or yang, tonify and/or move *chi*, calm the heart, or administer other related treatments. It should be remembered that menopause is a natural occurrence and that in many cultures where it is more accepted—even revered—it occurs symptom-free.

Acupressure treatment involves a variety of point-stimulation techniques that redirect the flow of energy in the body, and, in the process, prompt secretion of the body's painkilling chemicals. Acupuncture is based on the same principles as acupressure, but must be performed by a skilled professional with years of training (for more information, see "Acupuncture," Chapter Three).

Described below are various acupressure remedies for common menopausal complaints. Unless otherwise noted, you should press each acupressure point firmly but gently for two to three minutes, or until you feel relief. For further instructions on how to apply acupressure and precautions, see "Acupressure," Chapter Three.

While acupressure is a gentle, safe treatment when used properly, some precautions should be taken. You should never use acupressure as a *primary* treatment to relieve excessive bleeding, vaginal discharges, or undiagnosed pain, each of which can be an indication of serious illness requiring prompt medical care. Consult a physician first.

For Hot Flashes

- *Kidney 7:* You'll find this point just in front of the achilles tendon, about two inches above the tip of the inner anklebone.

- *Heart 6:* This point is located on the smallest-finger side of the hand, palm facing up, about a half-inch above the wrist crease on the inside of the tendon.

- *Gallbladder 20:* This point is situated on either side of the back of the neck below the skull in the depression between the trapezius and sternocleidomastoid muscles. See diagram at back of book.

- *Pericardium 6:* You can locate this point about three finger-widths from upper crease of the wrist on the inner forearm between the two tendons.

For Waning Sexual Interest

- *Conception vessel 4:* Feel for this point about four finger-widths directly below the bellybutton, or about two thumb-widths above your pubic bone.

- *Stomach 30:* This point is situated about two inches away from the midline of the abdomen on the upper border of the pubic bone.

- *Stomach 36:* This point is located on the calf, four finger-widths below the bottom of the kneecap, one finger-width on the outside of the shinbone. The point is on a muscle, so you'll know you're in the right place if you can feel it move when you flex your foot.

For Vaginal Dryness

- *Conception vessel 2:* This point is situated on the upper border of the pubic bone, in line with the bellybutton.
- *Large intestine 4:* You'll feel this acupressure point in the upper part of the web between the thumb and forefinger on the back of the hand.
- *Liver 2:* You'll find this point on the top of the foot on the web between the first and second toes near to the margin of the web.
- *Spleen 6:* You can find this point by placing four fingers above the ankle on the inside of the leg, right behind the shinbone.

For Insomnia or Depression

- *Liver 3:* This point is located on the top of the foot in the depression beyond the juncture of the metatarsal bones of the big toe and the second toe.
- *Anmian:* You'll find this point below the skull on the posterior edge of the mastoid, midway between gallbladder 20 (above) and the depression behind the earlobe.
- *Spleen 6:* Locate this point about four finger-widths up from the inside anklebone right behind the shinbone.
- *Pericardium 6:* You can locate this point about three finger-widths from upper crease of the wrist on the inner forearm between the two tendons.

- *Heart 7:* With the palm facing up, this point is located on the wrist crease on the smallest-finger side of the hand under the tendon. It is especially helpful in relieving emotional symptoms of anxiety and irritability.
- *Yintang:* You'll find this point between the eyes, right above the nose.

For Anxiety or Irritability

- *Liver 3:* This point is located on the top of the foot in the depression beyond the juncture of the metatarsal bones of the big toe and the second toe.
- *Large intestine 4:* You'll feel this acupressure point in the upper part of the web between the thumb and forefinger on the back of the hand.

AEROBIC EXERCISE

Aerobic exercise can be a wonderful elixir for the immediate discomforts of menopause as well as a strong ally against long-term health risks that can develop in later years. It may also reduce the severity of hot flashes, which are often worse in women whose bodies have difficulty with sweating. Increased activity causes the body to heat up and perspire to cool itself. Perspiration may help the body to better manage the dilation during a hot flash, thus reducing its impact. Aerobic exercise also causes the body to release its natural painkilling endorphins and enkephalins, which can relieve a range of menopausal complaints, from vaginal pain to irritability. But aerobic exercise also provides many preventive benefits: it lowers heart disease risk, improves circulation, decreases blood pressure, protects against heart disease, and lowers blood sugar.

Aerobic exercise can counteract the increased risk for heart disease that women over age fifty face by lowering risk in several ways. First, exercise causes increase of the HDL cholesterol, the "good" cholesterol that keeps the "bad" LDL cholesterol from clogging the arteries. Even walking at a leisurely pace of three miles per hour, five times per week, raises HDL cholesterol. This pace does not provide the aerobic benefits that are useful in lowering heart-disease risk even further, nor will it stimulate the body's natural painkillers, however. By exercising regularly so that your heart rate is within appropriate training levels (see chart on page 68), you can strengthen your heart muscle. Improved cardiovascular functioning means that the muscle will pump more blood through the body, and the body can better utilize oxygen and other nutrients. Together, these improvements reduce the workload on the heart, allowing it to work at a more restful rate. Finally, aerobic exercise lowers blood pressure, also common among middle-aged people, which raises risk of heart disease and stroke.

In addition to these benefits, exercise can help keep muscles toned and ward off fat, a condition that becomes more common during the middle years when metabolism slows. One third of all middle-aged women are estimated to be obese, and weighing 130 percent or more of your desired weight places you at increased risk for diabetes and heart disease.

In all, launching an exercise program may be the best investment of time you'll ever make! If you decide to make a go of exercise, it's best to start with a walking program and gradually increase your pace. For more information about how to establish a walking or running regimen, see "Aerobic Exercise," Chapter Three.

For another natural exercise remedy for menopausal complaints, see "Hatha Yoga."

AROMATHERAPY

Aromatherapy combines the strength of the essential oils found in plants with the powerful sense of smell to promote physiological and emotional benefits. A gentle yet effective ally during menopause, aromatherapy can be used to relieve a variety of ailments, from hot flashes to insomnia.

Listed below are suggested remedies for common menopausal complaints. Unless otherwise noted, you should notice results right away, and do not need to continue therapy after your condition is improved. For a preventive treatment for maintaining balance and health, see "Aromatherapy," Chapter Three.

For General Menopausal Complaints (Fatigue, Irritability, Hot Flashes)

Bath. Cypress is a vasoconstrictor; thus, it effectively counteracts the effects of hot flashes, which occur during vasodilation. Use three drops each of basil and cypress oils in a daily bath while the symptoms occur to soothe mind and body.

Massage. This massage will have an overall rejuvenating effect during menopause: Make an oil of two drops of thyme, rosemary, cypress, and basil oils in a carrier oil. Ask a friend to massage this into your abdomen, lower back, and the back of your neck, according to the following instructions:

First apply oil on the side you're working. Begin with the neck and, using one thumb, work down one side at a time, applying pressure at equal intervals. To massage the lower back, begin at the lower curve of the spine and, using both thumbs side by side, apply pressure about a half-inch away from the spine, working down one side of it. Use a fast movement for a stimulating effect and a slow movement for relaxation. Finish at the coccyx (the "tail" of the spine), then begin again, working down the other side of the spine. Try to apply pressure at the same intervals on each side. Apply oil to the other side of the body. To massage the abdomen, use the palm of your hand to rub in a clockwise motion.

For Insomnia

Bath. Lavender and neroli are gentle narcotics recommended for relieving mental and physical strain. Take a warm bath a half-hour before going to bed using six drops of either lavender or neroli oils.

Massage. Prepare a massage oil using two drops neroli, lavender, and melissa or petitgrain oils and apply to shoulders, solar plexus, and abdomen.

To Bring on Menstrual Period and Encourage Flow

Massage. Make a massage oil of one drop each of basil, chamomile, clary sage, juniper, lavender, marjoram, and rosemary. Apply to the lower back and abdomen.

For Emotional Upset See "Aromatherapy," Chapter Three.

BREATHING FOR RELAXATION

This relaxation technique is marvelous because it can be performed on the spot almost anywhere. It helps to counteract chronic stress, which increases risk for many diseases, including high blood pressure, elevated blood cholesterol, stroke, and heart attacks, all of which are concerns once we reach middle age.

Stress also can be an important influence on our experience of symptoms and illness. Thus, stress-fighting techniques like breathing can not only be a valuable ally in combating health risks but also in reducing menopausal discomfort and, in the process, enhancing our feelings of well-being and satisfaction during mid-life.

The best way to reduce stress is to interrupt our body's physiological reaction called the "fight or flight" response. Rapid, shallow breathing is one of the first signs of a stress response; thus, we can interrupt this response by breathing deeply and fully. To learn how to breathe healthfully, try the belly-breathing practice in "Breathing for Relaxation," Chapter Three.

HATHA-YOGA

Yoga can not only be a useful tool in counteracting many menopausal complaints, but can also be a wonderful anti-aging tool as well. According to yoga philosophy, it is the flexibility of a person's spine, not the number of years, that defines a person's age. Yoga is based on ancient Indian traditional beliefs that five "sheaths" of being are found in life. Imbalance of these sheaths—which include physical, mental, and spiritual energies and thoughts—results in disease. Most gynecological problems, including menopausal complaints, are seen as the manifestations of excess energies being released.

While the yoga positions called asanas can rebalance energies and eradicate disease, regular yoga practice can also reduce the impact of aging on the body. Such a program increases spine flexibility and removes tension from the body, important components of disease prevention. But hatha-yoga can also help to preserve muscle tone, firming up the skin, strengthening abdominal muscles, and preventing a double chin or flabby arms. Hatha-yoga has some other preventive benefits as well. In general, standing asanas strengthen the muscles of the legs, buttocks, abdomen, back, and shoulders. Strong muscles are instrumental in preserving good posture, preventing structural-related diseases and skeletal malformations. Strong abdominal muscles can help to maintain alignment of some of the internal organs and preserve muscle tone in the uterus, thus preventing a common condition called uterine prolapse (shifting) during the elderly years.

Treatment for excess energies involves practicing asanas throughout the month. (See Chapter Three for the following exercises.) For maximum effectiveness, first perform the belly-breathing practice (see "Breathing for Relaxation") and the practice meditation (see "Meditation"), then warm up with the sun salutation (see "Hatha-Yoga").

The asanas listed below can be helpful in preventing specific menopausal conditions. You should incorporate the positions you choose into your daily routine. Unless otherwise noted, most stretches should be held for only ten seconds initially. Gradually increase to two or even several minutes if it is comfortable.

Hatha-yoga is safe and effective and can also be used in conjunction with any other natural therapy. Some positions may exacerbate conditions like hypertension, however, so they should be avoided by people with these conditions. Be sure to take note of any precautions for each exercise.

To Strengthen Abdominal Muscles

Single-Leg Lifts.   Lie on your back with arms parallel to the trunk of the body. To the count of six, lift your left leg up about two feet from the floor, or as far as you can go without feeling discomfort. Do not bend your knee. Hold in position for a count of two, then lower again to a count of six. Repeat with the right leg, then perform the whole sequence again. At first, these may seem tough, but before you know it, they'll become easy. When you become proficient with single-leg lifts, try raising *both* legs at the same time.

Yoga Situp.   Lie on your back, and place your arms crisscross on your chest. To a count of three lift your head, neck, and shoulders several inches into the air. Hold this position for a count of three. Be sure that you feel this gently pulling from your abdomen. Then release your abdominal muscles as you sink to the floor at a count of three. Relax your abdominal muscles completely for a count of three. Repeat the sequence. Over time, lift your head, neck, and shoulders higher, to about eight inches from the floor. Increase your count to eight as well. Raising yourself incorrectly can cause neck strain, so be sure to let your abdominal muscles pull the rest of your body into the air.

Abdominal Rock.   Lie on your back with a pillow under your head and neck. Pull your knees in, bending them, so that feet are flat on the floor and only a few inches from the buttocks. With your knees together, move them to the right several inches and hold them there for a count of two. Swing them back to the center, holding for a count of two. Then swing to the left for a count of two. Repeat the exercise, but swing several inches further to each side. Gradually increase the hold to a count of ten. When you have mastered this practice, try holding your knees to your chest with your arms and then performing the exercise.

Bridge. This position is more advanced than the previous exercises, so try it after practicing them for several weeks. Lie on your back with your legs several inches apart and your arms parallel to the trunk of the body. Bend your knees, then lift your abdomen into the air as if a string from the bellybutton is pulling you up. Bend your arms and, with your elbows at each side of your chest, place your flattened palms underneath your body to brace it. Be sure that your shoulders remain on the floor. Hold the position for ten seconds, or as long as you can without feeling discomfort. To relax, release your hands and arms and let your abdomen sink into the floor and your knees straighten. Over time, increase the position to one or two minutes.

For Improved Musculoskeletal Strength and Good Posture

Free Pose. At first you may need to use a chair for help in holding this position, but with practice you can become quite proficient at this full-body strengthener. Stand up straight and tall, breathing deeply so that air fills your lungs. For balance, bring your hands together in front of your chest as if praying. Turn your right foot outward and bring the heel to touch the inner arch of your left foot. Reach down with your right hand, and lift your right foot to place the sole as high as possible against the left thigh. (Your right leg will form a triangle with the left leg.) Use a chair to steady yourself if necessary, but ultimately learn to balance yourself by placing all of your weight on your left foot. Focusing your gaze on a spot on the wall may help you to keep your balance. Hold the position for thirty seconds. Then repeat on the other side. Gradually increase time to several minutes. When you have mastered this, you may want to try a bigger challenge by holding the same position but with your arms raised above your head and palms together.

HERBS

During menopause, when the body is going through a physiological transformation, herbs offer a gentle treatment that will not compound discomforts. Standard allopathic treatment, estrogen replacement therapy, is often harsh and can cause very uncomfortable side effects, but herbs offer a natural form of replacement therapy. Other herbs promote relaxing and sedativelike qualities, so can be used to relieve a variety of other complaints during menopause, like achiness and vaginal pain.

Taking the herbs below in the recommended quantities should produce results almost immediately. Once results are achieved, stop taking the herb. In all cases, do *not* take the herb for longer periods or in greater doses than recommended. Herbs should not be taken while using aromatherapy or homeopathy, but can be combined with most other natural therapies. Also, you should consult with your regular health provider before undertaking any herbal therapy.

For more information on herbs and precautions, see "Herbs," Chapter Three.

Black Cohosh (*Cimicifuga racemosa* or *Macrotys actaeoides*). The roots of this plant, which belongs to the same family as the buttercup, were used by Native Americans and colonialists for gynecological remedies. This herb can relieve menstrual and menopausal discomfort by mimicking the female hormone estrogen. Decreased levels of the hormone estrogen during menopause are believed to be the cause of many complaints. For more information, see "Herbs," Chapter Three.

Feverfew (*Matricaria* or *Chrysanthemum parthenium*). Most of the news that has been spread about the leaves of this plant, a member of the same family as the daisy and the dandelion, are its remarkable effectiveness in suppressing migraine headaches. But menopausal women may also find it useful in lowering blood pressure.

Feverfew is believed to neutralize "bad" prostaglandins, the hormonelike chemicals in the body that are linked with high blood pressure. High blood pressure is one risk for heart disease, a concern for postmenopausal women. For more information, see "Herbs," Chapter Three.

Ginseng (*Panax quinquifolius* or *Panax ginseng*). The roots of this member of the ivy family have attracted the attention of healers and peddlers alike for centuries. With sister plants native to both China and the United States, ginseng has been credited with enough properties to make it highly sought after. Menopausal women can greatly benefit from this herb because it has several wonderful benefits that can lower heart-disease risk. Ginseng lowers levels of "bad" LDL cholesterol *and* raises amounts of the "good" HDL cholesterol that keeps the LDL cholesterol from clogging the arteries. Ginseng also has an anticlotting ability in the arteries, which reduces risk of heart disease and stroke. For more information, see "Herbs," Chapter Three.

Mistletoe (*Phoradendron serotinum*).   The leaves, berries, and twigs of this herb, most renowned as the Christmas "kissing" plant for those who walk under it, has another beneficial effect on the heart as well! Mistletoe lowers blood pressure, a risk factor for heart disease and stroke, making it useful for menopausal women, who are at increased risk for these conditions. This herb also may be useful for perimenopausal women because of its ability to promote menstruation, making it valuable for regulating the menstrual cycle. It is used widely in Europe in cancer therapy as a tumor-fighting agent.

Precautions: Mistletoe should only be used while you are under a physician's care. Because of its ability to slow the heart rate, it should be avoided by anyone with a history of heart disease or stroke. Because it is a uterine stimulant, it should be *avoided* by pregnant women. Mistletoe may cause a harmful reaction when taken simultaneously with a class of antidepressant drugs called MAO inhibitors. Do not give this herb to children or to elderly people.

Preparation: Under the care of a physician, you may develop an infusion by steeping one teaspoon of dried herb in one cup of boiling water for fifteen minutes. Drink no more than one cup per day. In a tincture, take only four drops each day.

Motherwort (*Leonurus cardiaca*).   The prized leaves, flowers, and stems of this member of the mint family can be quite useful for perimenopausal and menopausal women for several reasons. Motherwort may be unique— rarely does an herb known to be a uterine stimulant also have a tranquilizing effect. This herb may be useful for perimenopausal women because of its ability to promote menstruation, making it useful for regulating the menstrual cycle. Its tranquilizing effect can help to soothe the ills of perimenopause, not the least of which is sleep deprivation! Finally, motherwort has shown some ability to promote heart relaxation, to reduce clotting in the arteries, and to lower blood pressure, thus making it a helpful tool in lowering the risk of heart disease.

Precautions: Because motherwort is a uterine stimulant, it should be *avoided* by pregnant women. Because it may have anticlotting properties, it should be avoided by hemophiliacs or others with clotting disorders. It should also be avoided by those who are taking antihypertensive, cardiac, or sedative medications. Do not give this herb to children or elderly people.

Preparation: For an infusion, steep two teaspoons of the herb in one cup of boiling water for fifteen minutes. Drink no more than one and one-half cups each day. In a tincture, ingest no more than two teaspoons of this herb each day.

Red Clover (*Trifolium pratense*). While it has been touted for one hundred years primarily as a cancer treatment, the flower tops of this three-leafed herb also can relieve menstrual and menopausal discomforts because of its estrogenlike effects. For more information, see "Herbs," Chapter Four.

Vervain or Blue Vervain (*Verbena hastata*). An encyclopedic array of uses for this aspirinlike herb from the time of the ancient Egyptians, Greeks, and Romans to the present, make its leaves, flowers, and roots cherished. A species of this is available in Europe that is cousin to the U.S. variety. An anti-inflammatory agent and pain reliever, this herb can relieve a variety of minor discomforts related to menopause, from headache to achiness. But that's not all that makes vervain valuable. This herb may have the ability to promote menstruation, thus making it useful in regulating the menstrual cycle during perimenopause. Vervain also has a mild laxative effect. For more information, see "Herbs (for Osteoarthritis)," Chapter Nine.

HOMEOPATHY

The discomforts of menopause can often be subdued gently by the individualized healing actions of homeopathy. During menopause, women's lives can become unbalanced because of the physiological and emotional impact of hormonal changes. Homeopathy helps the body to regain balance to overcome such symptoms of discomfort by stimulating the immune system with substances that would produce a similar set of symptoms in a nonsufferer. Once the body's inherent healing powers are restored, women can regain a feeling of being centered and contemplate the road ahead in this most important passage of life.

If you are treating yourself, it's important to match your feelings and physical symptoms as closely as possible with the remedies listed below, just as a homeopath would. Unless otherwise noted, take a dose of 30c. For menopausal discomfort, take remedies no more than twice daily. *Stop* taking medication once symptoms begin to disappear. If your medication has no effect, it usually indicates that you have taken the wrong remedy. In that case, review your symptoms, and, being as specific as possible, match them to another remedy.

Homeopathy may be used in conjunction with some therapies like acupuncture, chiropractic, and hypnosis (Chapter Eight), or Psychotherapy (Chapter Two). But it should generally not be used simultaneously with aromatherapy or herbs because the former's essential oils may inactivate the homeopathic solution, as will coffee, alcohol, tobacco, perfumed cosmetics, and pungent household cleansers. It should also not be used as a substitute for traditional medical care for any serious ailment or condition.

For General Menopausal Discomforts (Hot Flashes, Emotional Upset, etc.)

- *Pulsatilla:* For changes in temperature—hot flashes and cold chills—with weepiness and insomnia, take this popular remedy.

- *Caulophyllum:* When emotional symptoms of nervousness and anxiety take over, use this remedy to calm down.

- *Cimicifuga:* When nervousness, irritability, and restlessness or insomnia take over, with a headache to boot, this may give you tremendous relief.

- *Lachesis:* Use this remedy when symptoms are worse after waking up, for hot flashes, headache, sweating, and tightness in the chest.

- *Sulphuric acid:* When hot flashes grow worse at night, moods are constantly changing, and fatigue persists, increasing after exercise, this remedy may be helpful.

- *Veratrum viride:* When hot flashes are very intense and are your primary symptom, try this aid.

- *Sanguinaria canadensis:* When intense hot flashes are accompanied by bad headaches, this may be your remedy.

For Insomnia

- *Valeriana officinalis:* When irritability and insomnia are your primary symptoms, take this to induce soothing and restful sleep.
- *Rhus toxicodendron:* When pain and discomfort lead to irritability and restlessness and pacing the floor at night, try this to calm your mind and body.

For Heavy, Irregular Periods

Note: This condition could be a warning sign that another more serious condition has developed (see Chapter Five and Chapter Eight).

- *China officinalis:* For menstrual periods that are sporadic and generate a headache, cramps, and light-headedness, this remedy can help you.
- *Ipecac:* When bleeding is profuse and accompanied by nausea, try this for relief.

For Emotional Symptoms

- *Sepia officinalis:* When discomfort leads to feelings of resentment and jealousy of others, and irritability, constipation, chilliness, and weakness are also symptoms, this remedy may be of great benefit.

HYDROTHERAPY

Hydrotherapy combines the metabolic effects of water with the restorative properties of heat and cold to improve our body's functioning and relieve pain. Water therapy is based on the premise that promoting action in one part of our body will create additional benefits in other parts as well.

There are many time-tested applications that are useful for soothing discomforts such as pelvic pain and enhancing relaxation during menopause. For example, the sitz bath, which relieves pelvic pain, is one of the oldest hydrotherapy techniques known.

For specific applications, see "Hydrotherapy," Chapter Four.

IMAGERY

Menopause is such an important and symbolic passage of a woman's life that celebrating the road ahead is in order. At this time of life, a woman has the maturity, confidence, and wisdom to embark on a new road and the freedom to do so. Visualization, a form of imagery, can be used to heighten self-fulfillment by envisioning what steps ahead you would like to take. It is especially helpful in relieving anxiety that you may feel during this period, perhaps about a new career move, new freedom from responsibility, or a new relationship. Relaxation imagery, in which we envision a soothing and peaceful scene, can also be helpful in this regard. And once you learn to relax, your composure will help you to better manage the stresses of everyday life. Besides reducing anxiety, relaxation can reduce the level of intensity with which women often experience menopausal discomforts. Try the relaxation imagery technique (see "Imagery," Chapter Three) twice daily to relax. If you are experiencing hot flashes, adapt the exercise to include some very stimulating images, or develop a scene in which a cool, chilly stream of water is flowing through your body, cooling it from the inside out. Don't forget to make the images as detailed and meaningful as possible to enhance imagery's effectiveness.

Imagery can be used in conjunction with any natural therapy, but offers its greatest advantages when combined with biofeedback (Chapter Two), hypnosis (Chapter Eight), and other relaxation techniques.

MASSAGE

Massage can be a wonderful tonic during menopause, not only because of its physical comfort, but also its emotional benefits. Massage can invigorate or relax us, depending on what techniques are used. The benefits of massage include improving circulation and releasing emotional tension that can lodge in our muscles. A restorative and soothing massage can offer women an opportunity to become focused in the present so that they can gain personal insight during this change of life.

The massage warmup will loosen tissue and relax the body to promote sleep, which can often be interrupted during perimenopause. It can also promote a feeling of emotional well-being during a difficult transition. Ask a helper to read the instructions and apply the techniques for you (see "Massage," Chapter Three).

Massage can be used in conjunction with any alternative therapy, and is often combined with acupressure, aromatherapy, and chiropractic. For additional applications, using essential oils, see aromatherapy.

MEDITATION

During menopause, women may find themselves distracted by everything from physical discomfort to psychological changes. Meditation provides a simple and quick technique for tuning out the noise so that women can get in touch with their inner selves and experience peace and tranquility. Meditation is the state of existing in the present without considering the concerns of tomorrow or even an hour from now. By relaxing during meditation, women are better able to manage concerns that otherwise would wear them down. In addition, reducing anxiety can have a wide array of health benefits, from reducing the risk of stress-related conditions and illnesses to minimizing menopausal discomforts. Try the practice meditation (see "Meditation," Chapter Three) twice daily to relax.

NUTRITIONAL THERAPY

During middle age, our bodies' nutritional needs begin to change. Our metabolism slows, and fewer calories are required. While the recommended calorie intake decreases, the recommended intake of most vitamins and minerals remains much as it was in early adulthood, except that protein and iron needs decrease slightly. Calcium needs may increase a great deal if you are at risk for developing osteoporosis (see Chapter Nine). Thus, with a constant nutrient requirement and reduced caloric needs, middle age is an important time to eat a diet of nutrient-dense foods.

Eating healthfully has other benefits as well. A lean and healthy diet can help postmenopausal women to counteract the risk of heart disease, which becomes equal to that of men. Weighing more than 130 percent of your recommended body weight puts you at increased risk.

High levels of cholesterol (over 200 milligrams per deciliter) can also contribute to the development of atherosclerosis, the buildup of fatty deposits in the coronary arteries that can lead to heart attack. Thus, eating foods that are low in cholesterol, the substance found in animal products, and reducing saturated fats, oils that can increase the body's cholesterol count, is very important. Eating foods that contain great amounts of saturated fats raise the blood cholesterol even more than eating foods high in cholesterol, like eggs, organ meats, and other animal products. But any fat can add weight to the body, and many studies link dietary cholesterol with increased risk for heart disease, so it's important to reduce intake of both cholesterol and fat.

Blood cholesterol readings include the "good" HDL cholesterol, which sweeps the "bad" LDL cholesterol from the arteries. In general, HDL levels should be about one third of total cholesterol levels. In other words, if your total cholesterol count is 160 milligrams, about 50 of those milligrams should be HDL cholesterol, and about 110 can be LDL cholesterol. Eating foods high in soluble fiber like fresh fruits and vegetables, oat bran, and legumes can lower LDL levels. Conversely, genetic factors, lack of exercise, cigarette smoking, and obesity can lower HDL levels.

Only about half of the fat from beef and other hoofed animals is saturated: poultry fat is slightly less saturated, while two thirds of fats from dairy products is saturated, but all animal products, of course, contain cholesterol. Fish oils, in contrast, are mostly polyunsaturated. Most saturated fats interfere with the removal of cholesterol from the blood, causing blood cholesterol levels to be high. Polyunsaturated and monounsaturated fats, however, lower blood cholesterol. In addition, cutting back on saturated fat will minimize damage caused by free radicals, destructive cells that weaken the immune system and can lead to disease.

Again, however, loading up on polyunsaturated fats, which keep cholesterol levels down, may not be wise. Some studies show that polyunsaturated fats may interact with oxygen to form free radicals as well. Thus eating a low-fat, low-cholesterol diet (your body can make all of the cholesterol it needs) that includes more of the unsaturated than saturated oils will make your body hum happily through middle age.

To be safe, most nutritionists recommend a diet containing 30 percent or less of total calories from fat, one third of which is taken from each group—polyunsaturated, monounsaturated, and saturated fat.

Evening-primrose oil is also very effective in lowering blood cholesterol and lowering blood pressure, two risks for heart disease. It's high in gamma-linolenic acid (GLA), which helps to synthesize the "good" prostaglandins that produce these healthful effects. You'll find it in capsule form at your local health-food store. Possible side effects include headaches and a feeling of lethargy. If these symptoms occur, discontinue use.

Besides paving a good-health road to the future, good nutrition can provide a safe and effective remedy for many discomforts associated with menopause. Many menopausal complaints are associated with dips in estrogen during perimenopause and the body's decreased synthesis of the hormone after menopause. By eating foods containing nutrients that enhance estrogen's effectiveness, we can maximize the effects of the remaining estrogen in our bodies and thereby minimize discomfort. Adequate amounts of vitamin B_6, vitamin E, vitamin C, folic acid, and PABA (para-aminobenzoic acid, a component of folic acid)—are all needed for estrogen production. Bee pollen, which contains all twenty-two amino acids used by the body, is also believed to promote the development of estrogen by the body. Unrefined whole grains are likewise believed to stimulate estrogen production.

In addition, eating foods that have estrogenlike properties can be helpful. See "Nutritional Therapy (for Breast Lumps)," Chapter Five.

Alone, vitamin E has shown promise for relieving common symptoms of menopause like fatigue, leg cramps, hot flashes, and vaginal dryness. Vitamin E is an anticoagulant so can promote blood flow in the body.

For natural food sources for these nutrients, see "Nutritional Therapy," Chapter Three.

Chapter Eight

Breast and Female Reproductive Cancers

Because of early detection methods, one out of two cancerous diseases are curable, and many more people learn to live productively with the disease for years. There are actually more than one hundred types of female reproductive cancers, each of which varies in growth rates and pattern, and each of which has a different impact on a person's health—and life. Having cancer can be as uncomplicated as finding a tumor in the body that does not produce any symptoms and can be removed quite easily. Such tumors are usually discovered through early detection methods like breast self-examination or a Pap smear, an examination of tissue taken from the uterus. If cancer is not detected early, however, it may grow larger and spread to other parts of the body.

While most types of female reproductive cancers can be detected early through screening methods, ovarian cancer is not often identified until in its advanced stages, when stomach upset and bloating are common. When any cancer becomes more advanced, it grows larger and can take over space needed by neighboring cells. Often it interferes with other cell functions by preventing them from doing their jobs. In addition, cancerous cells are usually dependent on other cells for nutrients since they cannot utilize energy well. Thus, cancer cells often weaken or destroy neighboring cells, causing some malfunctioning in the body because these cells are unable to fulfill their specialized function. Cancer cells can also metastasize, or spread to other parts of the body by hitching a ride on one of the body's two circulatory networks, the blood or the lymph system.

Our main defense against cancer is the immune system, the body's armory of defenses. The immune system protects us more than a thousand times each day against unfriendly invaders like cancer cells. It also fights off mobs of bacteria, gangs of viruses, bands of roving fungi or parasites, all of which try to wreak havoc in the body. With several lines of defense, the immune system identifies and develops a plan of attack against each type of intruder, then sets into motion its complex sequence of execution. Some cells flag invaders for destruction; others head directly to the invader and devour it; still others secrete hormones to produce a fever in the body to destroy invaders. Specialized cells "memorize" the unfriendly substance so that a future invasion can be thwarted immediately. If a few cancer cells are found in the body, they are usually destroyed by the immune system. When the body's immune system is weakened by illness, stress, or poor diet, for example, it can easily be overpowered by disease including cancer. In addition, because cancer cells can reproduce themselves quickly and are disguised by genetic mutations, they are often able to outnumber the immune system or evade its armed guards, which are unable to recognize its camouflage. Once cancer cells grow in rank, they can weaken the immune system, further lowering our defenses against cancer and other diseases.

Female breast and reproductive cancers affect almost a quarter of a million American women each year. Cancer of the breast, by far the most common female reproductive cancer, affects about 180,000 women each year. Breast cancer is usually found in breast tissue or in the lining of mammary gland ducts; if metastasized it may be found in lymph nodes of the armpit, or elsewhere in the body. Endometrial cancer, found in the lining of the uterus, the endometrium, makes up 90 percent of all uterine cancer and affects 32,000 women each year. Ovarian cancer, which affects 21,000 women each year, is perhaps the most risky cancer. Because the ovaries are concealed from view, ovarian cancer is more difficult to detect. Ovarian cancer is often found on the outer layer of the ovary, where it can spread quite easily to other organs in the abdomen and pelvis. Another female reproductive cancer, of the cervix, which is located at the opening to the uterus, affects about 13,500 women each year.

Genetic changes are believed to cause the development of reproductive and other cancers, although scientists are not sure exactly how these changes result in cancer. They do know that each cell manufactures nutrients that are useful to the organ that it serves, although each also contains about 50,000 genes and knows how to make all of the nutrients in the body. This information is stored in genetic material called DNA, and the genes in each cell single out parts of the DNA for the cell's use, giving it instruction about how to do its work—to repair and reproduce itself, for example. When several genes in a cell become flawed, the instructions become skewed, and a mutated cell called cancer is produced. Because these mutated cells lack important components that are necessary for operating efficiently, the cancer cells must rely heavily on neighboring cells for survival.

The nonstop growth that becomes harmful to the body during cancer is actually a necessary process during other stages of our life—during fetal development, adolescence, and to repair injured tissue. During cancer, this growth switch is somehow turned on—some scientists believe that a "suppressor gene" is the cause of cancer growth that must be turned off before cell proliferation occurs. Before that can happen, however, some cells of the body must undergo a transformation that changes their function from normal to abnormal. In other words, cells that function normally suddenly begin to act strangely, and begin to reproduce themselves in an odd design, missing some parts and perhaps making too many other parts. This step, called mutation, is believed to be caused by any number of factors, some of which are potent *mutators* and others which only promote mutation. Radiation exposure is an example of a mutator, while dietary factors and reproductive history are believed to promote the likelihood of cancer development but are not themselves mutators. Of course, we can inherit a mutated gene from our parents. Yet, even inheriting genes for cancer from your parents won't actually cause cancer, except for the rare exception of a cancer of the retina called retinoblastoma. Several lifestyle or environmental factors must also play a role in cancer development.

Reproductive history is another lifestyle factor affecting the development and growth of female reproductive cancers because of hormonal influences on the reproductive organs. Many clinicians believe that unopposed estrogen is a promoter of reproductive cancers, since late menopause and using estrogen replacement therapy, for example, which increase the body's exposure to estrogen, are considered risk factors for some reproductive cancers. Pregnancy has a protective benefit against some cancers like breast cancer because levels of estrogen that surge during gestation cause cells in the breast to mature and become specialized, or differentiated. Because breast cancer can only develop in cells that are undifferentiated, delaying childbirth or having no children increases the risk for developing this type of cancer because cells remain unprotected for a longer period of time. Thus, the risks for breast cancer include not having children or having a first child after age thirty. In addition, experiencing late menopause, being more than 40 percent overweight, being over the age of fifty, or having had a personal or family history of breast cancer increase breast-cancer risk. Silicone breast implants, while not known to be a direct cause of breast cancer can increase fibrous tissue that conceals breast lumps. Implants can also leak fluid, which may seep into a woman's lymph nodes and cause immune-system damage.

Conversely, early menopause, having children at an early age, and using oral contraceptives all protect against ovarian cancer. Women who have not given birth are twice as likely to develop ovarian cancer as those who have. Being over age sixty, more than 40 percent overweight, or having certain rare genetic disorders also increase the risk of developing ovarian cancer, and having had breast cancer doubles a woman's risk of developing this type of cancer.

And while the failure to ovulate protects against ovarian cancer, it *increases* the risk for endometrial cancer. Late menopause, a history of infertility, being more than 40 percent overweight, using estrogen replacement therapy, and using oral contraceptives all increase risk for endometrial cancer. Adding progesterone to the estrogen in hormone replacement therapy, however, can help to counteract the risk.

Unlike other reproductive cancers, cervical-cancer risk is largely attributed to lifestyle factors. Smoking cigarettes, having multiple sex partners, having intercourse at an early age and then having multiple sex partners, acquiring certain sexually transmitted diseases, and using oral contraceptives all increase risk of developing cervical cancer.

Despite the correlation between exposure to unopposed estrogen and the development of some reproductive cancers, cancerous tumors that develop may be responsive to other hormones like progesterone instead of or in addition to estrogen. Because hormones may stimulate the development or growth of some cancers and may hinder the growth of others, allopathic cancer specialists can perform a test called hormone-receptor assay to determine what effects certain hormones have on the tumor, which can then be helpful in treatment.

Other factors play a role in cancer development as well. Dietary factors are increasingly coming into the limelight as a method of cancer prevention and treatment. Certain fruits and vegetables contain vitamins called antioxidants that are believed to protect against substances in the body called free radicals, which may contribute to the development of cancer. Free-radical molecules cruise the body and attach themselves to cells to destroy them. They are produced during oxidation of saturated fats, a way for the body to make energy, and actually are necessary for some body functions. When the ranks of free radicals become excessive, however, they may prompt a chain reaction of damage to cells and alter the genetic material contained inside. Because free radicals can reprogram a cell's pattern of reproduction, many scientists believe that free radicals are the culprits that turn on the cancer switch of incessant reproduction. You can observe the destructive effects of free radicals when you slice open an apple and expose its flesh to oxygen—in a matter of minutes, it will deteriorate and become brown.

Environmental factors also contribute to cancer development. Radiation exposure is believed to directly contribute to the development of cancer, and it can cause all types of cancer but is a more prevalent cause of breast cancer than of any other female reproductive cancer. There are several types of radiation responsible for health problems. Alpha and beta particles cannot pass through the body's surface, so must be ingested or inhaled. High-frequency radiation found in X rays and low-frequency radiation found in radio and microwaves can penetrate the body and cause direct genetic damage. Radiation may be emitted from man-made sources such as dental and medical X rays and nuclear power plants, and from naturally occurring sources like radon, a gas that occurs during the natural breakdown of uranium in the soil. Having an X ray taken will not in itself cause cancer, but repeated X rays over a prolonged period of time or X rays from a faulty machine may do so.

Artificial low-level electromagnetic fields are also suspected to increase risk of certain types of cancer, including breast cancer. While some electromagnetic fields are natural—the earth and our bodies each possess them—almost anything plugged into an electrical circuit generates an artificial electromagnetic field while it is in operation that may be carcinogenic. Electromagnetic sources include personal-computer monitors, microwave ovens, electric power stations, refrigerators, televisions, electric blankets, and telephone lines. Of course, the strength of the electromagnetic field and the duration of exposure are both important factors in determining your level of risk. Household appliances generate much less risk and can be kept at a distance while in operation, as opposed to electric power lines, the field of which may remain strong for several hundred feet.

Environmental chemicals, another suspected contributor to the development of cancer and other diseases, thwart the removal of toxins from the body. We are exposed to toxins on a daily basis from plant and animal food sources. Animal food sources are often contaminated with hormones and antibiotics or even disease, and plant foods often contain pesticides and other harmful chemicals. Air and water pollution contribute a constant barrage of toxins to our bodies. All of these environmental toxins can penetrate our bodies and can overload the liver, which is responsible for filtering them from the blood. The liver is also responsible for the breakdown of estrogen to make it available for use by the body. Thus, when toxins overload the liver, it becomes overworked and is unable to perform all of its jobs efficiently. Excessive levels of estrogen cannot be released by the body until they are metabolized by the liver, so they circulate and eventually build up, and may contribute to the development or progression of estrogen-dependent tumors. A buildup of toxins can also have harmful effects on our health.

Thus, not one, but many factors may cause changes in the body before cancer can develop. And, while allopathic medicine focuses on treatment of cancer, natural therapies are useful in minimizing some of the risks that can lead to cancer development. Herbs can not only strengthen the immune system, but promote the removal of toxins from the body by strengthening the liver. Mind-body therapies promote relaxation and alleviate stress that can inhibit our immune system, and nutritional therapy can prevent some of the harmful effects of foods that can contribute to the development of cancer.

In addition, if cancer does develop, alternative therapies are quite helpful in relieving the side effects of allopathic treatments like surgery, chemotherapy, or radiation therapy. Natural therapies also can empower patients with the ability to affect their condition. This usually results in a feeling of well-being, which, in turn, may improve self-care and reduce symptoms. Herbs can strengthen the immune system that has been weakened by chemotherapy or radiation therapy. Mind-body therapies empower the individual for better self-care, promote relaxation, and minimize symptoms of illness and the side effects of treatment. Exercise can help eliminate fatigue, and it improves circulation of blood and lymph, often compromised by cancer treatment. Acupressure can help to rebalance energy and minimize symptoms, and nutritional therapy may help to prevent tumor growth.

Because of the powerful healing effects of both natural and allopathic medicine in fighting cancer, many patients develop a regimen that includes treatment from both systems of health care. When cancer patients are healed, there is no way to be sure which therapies were ultimately responsible. Thus, most natural-medicine practitioners recommend that a complex disease like cancer be treated by integrating conventional medicine to eradicate the cancer with alternative medicine for healing the person within.

If you find that you may be at risk for developing cancer, reduce your risks whenever possible. If cancer should develop, early detection is by far the most effective form of protection. If found early in their development, many cancerous tumors can be treated with few if any complications. More than 75 percent of all breast cancers are detected by women during self-examination. Several screening methods are available that can lead to early detection of female reproductive cancers, including the breast self-examination and mammography to detect breast cancer and the Pap smear, a scraping of tissue of the cervix and uterus, to detect cervical cancer. Some endometrial cancers are also detectable by the Pap smear, depending upon their location in the uterus. Ovarian cancer is not usually detectable by these routine screening methods and requires a full pelvic examination. If you are at risk for ovarian cancer, be sure to request regular, thorough pelvic examinations from your gynecologist. In addition, look out for any warning signs of cancer listed below. Because you won't necessarily see the symptoms of cancer described below until the disease is somewhat well-developed, it is very important to practice early detection methods.

WARNING SIGNS OF CANCER

Any of the following disturbances could be a warning sign of cancer, but also could be a symptom of a less serious condition. Irregular growth of cells in the body can be benign (noncancerous) as well as malignant (cancerous). A sluggish lymph system can cause the development of fluid-filled sacs called cysts in the reproductive organs, or surges in sex hormones during menopause may cause rapid cell division in the breasts that form lumps. Such cell growths are harmless and often disappear on their own, but natural therapy may also be used to alleviate them. (For more information, see Chapter Five). Certain irregular growths are suspected to be precursors to cancer, however, such as certain sexually transmitted diseases are believed to heighten risk for cervical cancer, so be sure to get them checked out by your physician.

If you detect any of these symptoms, ask your doctor to investigate them.

- *Breast cancer:* pain or soreness of the nipple; skin irritation or scaliness; a lump, thickening, swelling, dimpling, or hollow. The skin around a tumor can sometimes appear stretched and shiny with enlarged pores. An increased number of blood vessels may be visible.

- *Cervical or endometrial cancer:* an abnormal vaginal discharge or bleeding in between menstrual periods or following menopause.

- *Ovarian cancer:* distension of the abdomen, caused by the buildup of fluid. Unfortunately, these symptoms are not apparent until the cancer is in advanced stages. Persistent digestive disorders may also be an indication of ovarian cancer.

ACUPRESSURE/ACUPUNCTURE

When cancer occurs in the body, acupuncture can be quite helpful in counteracting the side effects of chemotherapy and radiation by strengthening the body. Acupuncture can alleviate such complications by normalizing *chi* flow throughout the body. Acupuncture is also very useful in minimizing the side effects of surgery. Before surgery, treatment can build up *chi* and thus reduce the trauma of surgery. After surgery, acupuncture can be very effective in promoting recovery by rebuilding *chi*. In addition, treatment can restore the flow of *chi* by promoting the healing of scars so that *chi* can reinsert itself into meridians that have been cut by surgery.

Treatment involves a variety of point-stimulation techniques to strengthen overall *chi* and, in the process, strengthen the body's healing capacity.

While acupuncture is a gentle, safe treatment when used properly, you should never use acupuncture as a *primary* treatment for cancer. Be sure to obtain primary cancer care from a licensed physician.

For Nausea

- *Pericardium 5:* You can find this point on either forearm, four finger-widths above the center of the inner wrist crease between the tendons.

- *Pericardium 6:* You can locate this point about three
  finger-widths from upper crease of the wrist on the
  inner forearm between the two tendons.

BREATHING FOR RELAXATION

This deep-breathing technique helps to counteract the
stress that may increase our susceptibility to cancer and
has been linked with an increased risk for many diseases,
including high blood pressure, elevated blood cholesterol,
stroke, and heart attacks. Our body's physiological experience of stress causes secretion of adrenal hormones,
which, when prolonged, can suppress the immune system.
A weakened immune system is not able to perform its vital
role in fighting off diseases, including cancer.

Deep breathing has other benefits as well. Its relaxing
effects can reduce anxiety stemming from having cancer,
which, in turn, can help to minimize your experience of
pain and discomfort related to the disease or its treatment.
It helps to stimulate the toxin-fighting lymph system.
Often a side effect of chemotherapy or other cancer treatment is that lymph is unable to circulate through the body
without exercise, deep breathing, or other stimulation. Because deep breathing can be a valuable ally in combating
health risks and reducing pain and discomfort, it may enhance our feelings of empowerment during illness. This
can result in a feeling of overall well-being and, as a result,
better self-care.

We can avert our body's reaction to stress, called the
"flight or fight" response, by learning to breathe fully and
deeply. Rapid, shallow breathing is the first sign of this
response. Try the belly-breathing practice in "Breathing
for Relaxation," Chapter Three.

EXERCISE

Experts believe that exercise may play a role in preventing cancer, just as it does in preventing heart disease—the more you exercise, the less chance you have of getting cancer. Some studies have shown that women athletes have significantly less incidence of cancers of breast and reproductive organs. This may be because exercise provides a host of benefits. It lowers levels of circulating estrogen in the body, high levels of which correlate with increased incidence of some cancers. By exercising regularly, you are less likely to become overweight, a risk factor for developing endometrial and breast cancer. In addition, exercise improves the circulation of vital nutrient-rich blood to all parts of the body. Blood cells carry not only oxygen but other valuable nutrients, keeping the cells well-nourished and the body healthy. One type of physical activity, aerobic exercise, increases the body's need for oxygen; and high levels of oxygen can have a negative effect on cancer cells. Exercise can also help to alleviate stress, which can play a role in suppressing the body's immune system. Finally, exercise helps to move toxin-fighting lymph through the body. Often lymph is unable to circulate without exercise or deep breathing or some other form of stimulation.

Cancer patients, who may benefit from exercise or physical fitness most, are typically not involved in them. Despite the many benefits of exercise, rehabilitation for cancer patients usually involves some form of physical therapy, but not physical activity. While chemotherapy and radiation therapy often sap your energy level, physical exertion can help to restore it. By developing a modified exercise program with your physician, you can also counteract other side effects of treatment. Exercise produces natural painkilling chemicals that can minimize pain and discomfort of both the disease and its treatment. Physical activity can reduce nausea and minimize fluid retention in the limbs, often a result of a poorly draining lymph system following cancer treatment. Exercise can also reduce levels of circulating estrogen, and thus may be helpful in slowing growth of a tumor that is estrogen-dependent. And, of course, a moderate workout can minimize your experience of anxiety and promote a feeling of well-being.

Finally, regular exercise can be a valuable tool for women with breast or other reproductive cancers to regain body acceptance after surgery or another invasive treatment.

If you are a cancer patient, it's important to consult your doctor about when and how much to exercise, because chemotherapy, for example, can sometimes cause heart irregularities, which can become exacerbated with exertion. Thus, most physicians and exercise physiologists recommend waiting at least one day after chemotherapy before exercising.

If you have cancer or want to help to prevent it, there are many types of physical activity from which you can benefit. Aerobic exercise offers an exceptional number of wonderful health benefits and can be performed at your own pace and at your convenience. It also provides many preventive benefits: it lowers heart-disease risk, decreases blood pressure, and increases the "good" HDL cholesterol that protects against heart disease and lowers blood sugar. If you decide to make a go of aerobic exercise, it's best to start with a walking program and gradually increase your pace. For more information about how to establish a walking or running regimen, see "Aerobic Exercise," Chapter Three.

HERBS

Natural herbs are effective and gentle, an important consideration during cancer when conventional treatment can have a harsh effect on the body. If you are undergoing cancer treatment, be sure to consult with your physician before taking any herb.

Herbs offer several benefits for the prevention and treatment of cancer that complement allopathic treatment. Herbs can be helpful in strengthening the body's liver, which is responsible for filtering toxins from the body, synthesizing valuable nutrients, and making the body's hormones available for use by the body. Some herbs have estrogenlike properties that may make them useful in counteracting the effects of estrogen-dependent tumors. This is because herbs supply a natural form of estrogen that is less potent than the body's estrogen. If you ingest these herbs, the body will absorb the gentler estrogen and release the stronger estrogen from the body (see Chapter Five). Herbs can be a helpful adjunct in counteracting the side effects of chemotherapy or other conventional cancer treatment by strengthening the body's immune system, which is weakened by treatment. Some herbs are believed to fight tumor growth.

Going to an herbalist can heighten benefits. A Chinese herbalist, of course, will treat you with a completely different criteria, based on a diagnosis using traditional Chinese medical principles and provide you with herbs that are not generally available to the public. (For more information, see "Oriental Medicine," Chapter Two.) In addition, an herbalist can diagnose complex mixtures of herbs that synergize to form healing effects specific to your condition.

Taking the herbs below in the recommended quantities should produce results almost immediately. Once results are achieved, stop taking the herb. In all cases, do *not* take the herb for longer periods or in greater doses than recommended below.

Herbs should not be taken while using aromatherapy or homeopathy, but can be combined with most other natural therapies.

For more information on healing herbs, see "Herbs," Chapter Three.

Alfalfa (*Medicago sativa*). The leaves of this member of the pea family appear to provide many health benefits, from lowering blood cholesterol, a risk for heart disease and stroke, to reducing cancer-causing substances in the body. Alfalfa is believed to contain substances that snatch up bits of carcinogenic material and escort them from the body, thereby decreasing the body's exposure to harmful substances.

Preparation: For an infusion, steep two to three teaspoons of dried leaves in a cup of boiling water for ten minutes. Do not drink more than two cups per day.

Precautions: Some evidence suggests that alfalfa may induce anemia, so do not drink more of this herb than is recommended. Anemic women should stay away from alfalfa. Do not give this herb to children. Elderly people should begin with a small dosage and gradually increase it. Do *not* eat the seeds of this plant because they contain toxic substances that, in large amounts, have been linked with blood-clotting disorders, infection, and lupus disease. Other substances in the seeds may promote menstruation and cause miscarriage, thus pregnant women should *avoid* alfalfa seeds as well.

Chaparral (*Larrea divaricata* or *L. tridentata*). The twigs and new leaves of this member of the same family as the star-thistle probably deserve its nickname, "stinkweed," but that's not chaparral's most notable quality.

Chaparral may be useful for preventing cancer because it contains a chemical that destroys some of the free radicals that cause cell damage in the body. Chaparral may also have the ability to slow down or decrease tumor growth, although this fact has not been well-documented.

Precautions: If you have cancer, use chaparral *only* under the supervision of your physician. Chaparral has been shown to cause kidney and lymph problems in animals. Therefore, those with kidney or lymph problems should avoid this herb. Pregnant or breastfeeding women should avoid this herb. Similarly it should not be given to children. Elderly people should begin with a low dose and gradually increase it.

Preparation: For an infusion, steep three teaspoons of dried leaves and twigs to about one and one-half quarts of water for forty-five minutes. Drink no more than four cups per day.

Echinacea (*Syzgium aromaticum* or *Eugenia caryophyllata*). The roots of this plant, a member of the same family as the dandelion, were once treasured by Native Americans. Echinacea was then discovered by Europeans, who use this herb to fortify the immune system. Americans have since rediscovered that echinacea contains natural antibiotics effective in warding off a range of invaders that can cause everything from colds and flu to yeast infections to fungus. Echinacea may be useful for preventing cancer because it increases the number of infection-fighting white blood cells in the body. This ability may make it valuable for cancer patients receiving radiation therapy, which lowers the white blood cell count, making patients particularly prone to infection or illness.

Precautions: If you are a cancer patient, use this herb *only* under the supervision of a physician. Echinacea does not commonly cause side effects except for a harmless tingling of the tongue. However, if you should experience any discomfort or pain from its use, discontinue use immediately, and consult your physician. Pregnant women should not take echinacea, and it should not be given to children. Elderly people should take a small dose and gradually increase it.

Preparation: For a decoction, steep three teaspoons of dried root in a cup of boiling water for twenty minutes. Drink no more than two cups per day.

Ginseng (*Panax quinquifolius* or *Panax ginseng*). The roots of this member of the ivy family have attracted the attention of healers and peddlers alike for centuries. With sister plants native to both China and the United States, ginseng has been credited with enough properties to make it highly sought after. It is also difficult to grow, making it rather expensive. However, ginseng has been shown to provide several benefits that can help middle-aged women counteract heart-disease risk. Ginseng may also be useful to cancer patients because it has been shown to minimize white blood cell loss that results from radiation therapy, an effect that can make the patient prone to developing infection or illness. In addition, ginseng may have the ability to slow down or decrease tumor growth, although studies are inconclusive. This herb also helps the liver to remove toxins from the body, which promotes overall health and prevents disease by minimizing toxic buildup. For more information, see "Herbs," Chapter Three.

Milk Thistle (*Carduus marianus*). This herb has been used by Europeans as a method of enhancing the functioning of the liver. It makes a wonderful liver-cleanser and promoter. The liver is responsible for filtering toxins from the blood. If the liver becomes overworked, unfiltered toxins are stored in the body, and a buildup of them can have harmful effects on our health. Milk thistle can also be helpful in promoting liver metabolism that is often compromised by chemotherapy or other conventional cancer treatments.

Precautions: Do not give this herb to elderly people or children. Pregnant women should *avoid* it.

Preparation: Steep one teaspoon of dried herb in one cup of boiling water for fifteen minutes. Drink no more than three cups per day. Another way to enjoy milk thistle is to soak the dried herb in water overnight, mince it in a food processor, and add about one teaspoon of it to cereal or to soups.

Turmeric (*Curcuma longa*). The roots of this member of the same family as ginger are prized by those with arthritis for their ability to reduce pain and inflammation. But turmeric may also be helpful in rejuvenating the liver and protecting it from damage caused by conventional cancer treatment. Studies involving liver-damaging drugs have demonstrated its protective effect. According to one study, turmeric may have a tumor-fighting property as well. For more information, see "Herbs (for Osteoarthritis)," Chapter Nine.

Mistletoe (*Phoradendron serotinum*). The leaves, berries, and twigs of this herb are renowned for their use in Christmas customs, but they are more valuable for their beneficial effect on cancer patients. These benefits of mistletoe have been well-documented in Europe, where it is used in chemotherapy to help fight cancer by slowing down tumor growth. Mistletoe may also help to counteract the effects of radiation therapy, which is known to reduce the amount of infection-fighting white blood cells in the body, by promoting the rapid growth of those white blood cells. For more information, see "Herbs," Chapter Seven.

Five-Herb Anticancer Fighter. Herbs have the unique ability to work synergistically to promote healing effects. Since their healing actions are unique, developing a mixture with a desired effect takes dedication and time. This blend of herbs has withstood the test of time as a potent tumor fighter. To make an infusion, steep one teaspoon of each of the following herbs in a quart of boiling water for thirty minutes. Drink no more than two cups per day: *chaparral* (described above), *echinacea* (described above), *juniper berries (Juniperis communis)*, *nettles* (Chapter Five) and red clover (Chapter Four).

HYPNOSIS

Hypnosis combines the healing images of the mind's eye with the power of the subconscious to promote healthy benefits. Hypnosis has been used for clinical applications since the late 1700s and remains an effective therapeutic tool today. Despite its association with the mysterious and suspenseful, hypnosis is a well-known mind-body technique for focusing our mind so that we can relax or control certain behaviors. A popular image of hypnosis—the hypnotized person on a stage clucking like a chicken—depicts a unique state produced by hypnosis, suggestibility. If you were to become fully hypnotized, you would be quite aware of your actions and would most likely be quite *willing* to perform certain actions if requested to do so. This phenomenon of suggestibility is enhanced by the highly focused state of the mind, because you are not distracted by thoughts.

Hypnosis utilizes the power of your mind to focus on a

particular thought or idea while disassociating from other sensations, thoughts, or occurrences. You experience disassociation when, for example, you wear jewelry. When you first don a necklace, you will be aware of the feeling of its heaviness around your neck. But as soon as your thoughts turn to something else, you will be unaware of any sensation against your skin, perhaps until you remove it. While clinicians aren't sure exactly why we become acquiescent during hypnosis, many believe it is because we are tapping into our subconscious mind, which then sends powerful messages to our conscious mind.

Regardless of why hypnosis works, imagine the potential health benefits that can be achieved when participants are willing to dispense with tired and unhealthy behaviors just by being asked! With your mind as the tool, there are many techniques for promoting health benefits and many ways in which to achieve them. For example, hypnosis can be used to curb compulsive behavior, relieve stress, or alleviate symptoms of pain. We can use a variety of techniques, from imagery to hand levitation, to induce this state of focused awareness. During hypnosis, we may be asked to hold images in our mind that are tranquil and serene to promote physiological and emotional relaxation. Similarly, we may visualize that health and vitality are being restored to our bodies to promote psychological well-being, which can have an effect on reducing symptoms of illness. Hypnosis has advanced applications as well. It has been used as an anesthetic during surgery for those who are allergic to anesthesia or reluctant to use it.

Hypnosis can be very helpful in relieving the discomforts associated with cancer or its treatment. It can also be helpful in alleviating some of the anxiety and stress that can be associated with having a disease that affects so many areas of our lives. Stress can be an important influence on our experience of symptoms and illness. Thus, stress-fighting techniques like hypnosis can not only be a valuable ally in combating health risks but also in reducing overall discomfort and, in the process, enhancing our feelings of well-being during illness. Through hypnosis, you can learn to transform the feeling of anxiety or pain into some other feeling, tune it out, and turn your attention to something else.

Because of its powerful nature, hypnosis may create benefits that last long after a hypnosis session. But you can enjoy benefits during the hypnosis session as well. For example, you can alleviate symptoms of pain under hypnosis by visualizing that you are floating in air while receiving chemotherapy or radiation therapy or during recovery—at whatever time is most uncomfortable. Once you become more advanced, you can hypnotize yourself easily while taking some treatments or during recovery. During this hypnosis session, you can visualize that you are floating in mid-air, thus minimizing the pain or discomfort that you feel. In lieu of floating in mid-air, you can imagine that you are doing something very enjoyable and feeling quite pleasant, or quite simply, you can visualize that you are numb and not feeling any pain! Not only will you reduce sensations of pain, but also feel less anxious about your condition in the long run, which, in turn, can minimize your symptoms.

While many prefer to visit a professional psychotherapist or hypnotist for initial hypnosis, self-hypnosis is possible for achieving light but effective states of trance. However, if you are having difficulty hypnotizing yourself or you want to achieve a deeper trance, you could benefit from the services of a professional hypnotist. Many psychotherapists are skilled in hypnosis, or if not, they can probably refer you to a trained hypnotist. For hypnosis involving pain relief, it is best to consult a professional hypnotherapist. Pain is the body's warning sign that dysfunction may be occurring, and if you suppress pain when it is a signal from the body, you could endanger yourself. Similarly, consult a professional if you decide to incorporate pre-hypnotic suggestions into your technique for reinducing hypnosis, for example. Such techniques can be hazardous if you are unclear about how or when you will awaken again. In all cases, the hypnotic state should not last any longer than five minutes to prevent you from falling into a natural sleep before awakening from hypnosis.

Below is a practice self-hypnosis exercise that you can try. The easiest way to hypnotize yourself is by, first, reading this exercise several times so that your mind has an image of how the body and mind will respond during hypnosis. Allow long pauses between sentences. You are putting the hypnotic suggestion into your mind so that, when you hypnotize yourself, you will not have to think about what to do. Thinking consciously will break the hypnotic state. Because a hypnotic state does not dull awareness, you may not be aware that you are under hypnosis; only the state of willingness produced actually indicates whether or not you are hypnotized.

Self-Hypnosis Exercise

Sit comfortably in a chair. Select a spot on the wall in front of you or on your ring, and keep your eyes focused on the spot. If your eyes wander, bring them back to the same spot. As you look at the spot, your eyes are becoming tired and your mind and body are beginning to feel tired, in need of rest and relaxation. Your eyes are growing tired of staring at the spot and your body and mind too would like some peace, some rest. The spot is harder to focus on now because it is becoming fuzzy and it sometimes appears as if it's moving. But you must keep your eyes on the spot until you are ready to relax. Your eyelids are beginning to become heavy and they are beginning to close on their own. It's okay to close them now. Your mind and body want to relax completely. Your breathing is slowing down now. It's growing deeper and slower. Deeper and slower. Your whole body is beginning to feel light, but you won't fall asleep. You only feel peaceful, very peaceful and calm. Your whole body is feeling buoyant, as if it could float. Feel the weightlessness in your toes—your small toes and your big toes, in your ankles and all around your calves. Your knees feel feathery and light. Your thighs, too, are feeling as if they are going to lift off the floor at any minute. As your body becomes lighter, you feel more relaxed and peaceful. Your buttocks and hips are feeling light now, too. Feel the buoyancy flow through your abdomen and up your chest. You're feeling quite relaxed, without any cares in the world now. Your back is so light it can hardly stay down. Feel the lightness of your shoulders and your arms . . . all the way to the tips of your fingers. You are feeling deeply relaxed, without any concerns. Your neck is as light as a feather. So is your face and your head. The top of your head feels like a balloon about to lift into the air. Your whole body weighs less than a single feather, light enough to lift off the ground. You're floating in mid-air now.

[Now give yourself constructive suggestions about relaxation, pain relief, or improved health.] In a few moments, you will open your eyes. Before doing so, your body will gently return to its original position and no longer float. When you open your eyes, you will feel completely relaxed and restored, yet very alert.

IMAGERY

During illness, we sometimes feel like we have little control over our lives. Imagery helps us to regain some autonomy by providing us with an opportunity to reduce the pain and discomfort associated with cancer. By envisioning how we would like to manage our illness and treatment, we can also shape our self-care. Such techniques can greatly improve the quality of life for cancer patients, enhancing well-being and allowing them to find peace and meaning in their lives.

Imagery has another application for cancer patients—envisioning cancer being eradicated from their bodies. While there is no scientific evidence that such a technique works, there have been enough cases of spontaneous remission by cancer patients who practice alternative medicine to promote inquiry as to the cause of remission. Try the relaxation imagery technique (see "Imagery," Chapter Three) twice daily to relax. If you are experiencing great emotional difficulty or physical discomfort, adapt the exercise to include some very stimulating images, or develop a scene in which your cancer is being healed. For example, visualize that cancer cells wave the white flag and are swept from the body by triumphant immune-system cells. Don't forget to make the images as detailed and meaningful as possible to enhance imagery's effectiveness.

Imagery can be used in conjunction with any natural therapy but offers its greatest advantages when combined with biofeedback (Chapter Two), hypnosis, and other relaxation techniques.

MASSAGE

Massage is used as a nurturing tool in many holistic cancer-treatment programs. Besides its soothing effect, a massage can nurture self-esteem and restore acceptance of the body if invasive treatments like surgery or radiation therapy have made you feel estranged from or critical about your body. Massage helps you to mentally reconnect the parts of your body, making you feel whole again. Massage can also activate a sluggish lymphatic system caused by chemotherapy or radiation therapy. Often lymph is unable to move through the body without exercise or some other form of stimulation.

The massage warmup will loosen tissue and relax the body while providing many benefits. Ask a helper to read the instructions and apply the techniques for you (see "Massage," Chapter Three).

Massage can be used in conjunction with any alternative therapy, and is often combined with acupressure (Chapter Three) and aromatherapy and chiropractic (Chapter Four).

MEDITATION

Meditation, a quiet state of mindful awareness, is another valuable component of many cancer-treatment programs. Meditation helps to achieve a state of deep physiological and emotional relaxation that is essential in restoring the body's ability to heal itself during cancer. Meditation also offers an opportunity to quiet our minds during periods of emotional stress, episodes of which we may experience during illness. Cancer can affect all aspects of a patient's life, and becoming focused on it instead of on you, while a natural tendency, can limit your maximum healing potential. By quieting your mind through meditation, you can alleviate some of the anxieties of cancer, address your emotional and physical needs, and restore some balance to your life. Relaxation can also help to minimize the symptoms of illness. Try the practice meditation (see "Meditation," Chapter Three) twice daily to relax. If you are experiencing great discomfort, try to observe anxious thoughts that accompany pain and let go of them. You may find that daily meditation gives you a new perspective on life, helping you to take it one day at a time.

NUTRITIONAL THERAPY

The role that diet and environmental factors play in cancer development is demonstrated time after time when immigrants from other countries develop the same health risks as people in their new homeland. For example, immigrants from Japan, where rates of stomach cancer are high and rates of breast cancer are considerably lower than in the United States, develop U.S. cancer risks after living here for several generations.

In recent years, certain foods have been discovered to go a long way toward fighting cancer by strengthening the body's immune system, destroying free radicals that can kill our cells and cause disease, and speeding up the process of eliminating carcinogenic substances from the body. In general, a diet high in fibrous fresh fruits, vegetables, and whole grains, and low in fat, sodium, and refined sugar, is recommended to promote health and to reduce the risk for a wide range of cancers. A high-fat diet was once believed to increase the risk of breast cancer, but now obesity and excessive calorie intake, rather than fat consumption alone, are believed to contribute to the development of breast cancer. Being 40 percent or more overweight increases risk for developing breast, ovarian, and uterine cancers, another good reason to add fiber and reduce fat in the diet.

Fruits and vegetables, as well as whole grains, provide another health benefit as well. Antibiotics, hormones, and toxins that exist in animals are passed on to us when we ingest them as a source of protein. Pesticides and chemical additives are abundant in many plant foods. All of these toxic materials enter our body and can have harmful effects, leading to disease. Thus, one way of reducing the impact of toxins on the body is speeding their elimination from it. Fruits, vegetables, and whole grains can move foods through the body three times faster than nonfibrous foods.

Promoting the health and metabolism of the liver, which is responsible for filtering toxins from the blood, may also be helpful in reducing toxins in the body and reducing the progression of certain estrogen-dependent tumors by reducing estrogen levels in the body. The liver is responsible for the breakdown of estrogen to make it available for use by the body. When we overwork the liver, it is unable to process estrogen efficiently, and excessive levels of estrogen circulate in the body. Because the body cannot release this form of estrogen until it is metabolized by the liver, it builds up and can contribute to a host of conditions, including female cancers. For more information, see Chapter Five.

Another way of minimizing cancer risk or progression is by incorporating cancer-fighting antioxidants into our diet. Each day, we each consume carcinogens in virtually every food substance. Since the 1980s it has been documented that all plant foods contain small amounts of carcinogenic substances. The reason we all don't get cancer is because plants also contain small amounts of anti-oxidant material. Anti-oxidants are substances that counteract the destructive effects of free radicals in the body. Free radicals are harmful substances that cruise the body, destroying cells, which can lead to disease. Thus, eating fruits and vegetables that contain antioxidants can help to tip the scales in our favor.

The vitamins and minerals listed below play a specific role in counteracting cancer. Some attack and neutralize the free-radical molecules; others are necessary to promote healthy functioning of the body's immune system, the body's first line of defense against cancer. Each nutrient plays a different role in preventing damage, so it's important to eat foods that are high in each of these nutrients to ensure protection. In addition, cutting back on saturated fat will prevent free-radical damage. Some studies show that polyunsaturated fats may also interact with oxygen to form free radicals. Until study results become conclusive, most nutritionists recommend a diet containing 30 percent of total calories from fat, one third of which is taken from each group—polyunsaturated, monounsaturated, and saturated fat. For cancer patients, the amount of daily calories from fat that are recommended may be even less, as low as 10 percent. For more information on fats, see "Nutritional Therapy," Chapter Seven. For a list of natural food sources of these nutrients, see "Nutritional Therapy," Chapter Three.

Vitamin A

The precursor to vitamin A, beta-carotene, is found in plants, and may provide preventive and therapeutic benefits for cancer patients because it searches for and destroys free radicals found in cells and molecules. Vitamin A is also believed to be effective in counteracting epithelial-cell cancers, which include most reproductive cancers. Some studies suggest that diets rich in vitamin A and fiber reduce the risk of ovarian cancer as well. Vitamin A is given to cancer patients in high doses in many cancer-treatment programs. However, do not ingest high doses of vitamin A except under the supervision of a physician. Excessive amounts of this vitamin are stored in the body and can be toxic. Large amounts of beta-carotene, on the other hand, found only in plants, are not toxic, although they may turn the skin an orange-yellow color.

Vitamin C

Vitamin C goes to work repairing the molecular damage caused by free radicals, which impair cell functioning. It also prevents oxidation of fatty foods by absorbing free radicals and ushering them from the body. In addition, vitamin C can increase the production of chemicals in the immune system that fight viruses and can boost the power of the immune-system cells that devour invaders. Vitamin C is also a catalyst for the formation of "good" pros- taglandins, which are believed to regulate tumor growth (see "Nutritional Therapy," Chapter Four). Some research indicates that Vitamin C is useful in preventing breast and cervical cancer.

Vitamin E

Another antioxidant, vitamin E protects against free-radi- cal damage in a unique way. Because vitamin E needs fat to become available for use by the body, it heads directly for cell membranes, which are typically high in fatty acids. There it protects the cell membrane from oxidation by sacrificing itself when free radicals approach. By saving the cell membrane, vitamin E causes cells to live much longer. Vitamin E increases the number and effectiveness of some types of immune-system cells. In concert with selenium, vitamin E can help to change cancer cells back to normal cells.

Vitamin K

Vitamin K has been shown to kill cancer cells of the breast and ovaries in laboratory tests.

Magnesium

The macro mineral magnesium is necessary for the production of "good" prostaglandins, which are believed to slow tumor growth.

Selenium

Another valuable nutrient in counteracting chronic disease, the trace mineral selenium preserves cell membranes by prompting toxic wastes like free radicals to leave the body. Selenium also contains an enzyme that deactivates free radicals, rendering them harmless. In concert with vitamin E, selenium increases the production of certain immune-system cells.

Zinc

Zinc is a partner with an important enzyme that fortifies cells and protects them from free-radical damage. Zinc also boosts the activity of infection-fighting white blood cells in the immune system.

B-Complex Vitamins

While all of the B-complex vitamins are essential for the proper functioning of the immune system, vitamin B_6 and vitamin B_{12} are particularly important for its development and fortification. Vitamins B_3 and B_6 are necessary for the production of "good" prostaglandins, which are believed to regulate tumor growth. Folic acid plays a role in preventing free-radical damage. A deficiency of folic acid has been linked with cervical cancer, so ensuring adequate amounts of foods containing this nutrient in the diet can provide preventive benefits.

Copper

The trace mineral copper is believed to fight the side effects of radiation. Some studies suggest that copper may be helpful in slowing tumor growth.

Some Cancer-Fighting Foods and Substances

The following substances are known cancer-fighters. Just adding a "dose" of them to your daily diet can provide wonderful preventive and therapeutic benefits.

- *Apples:* The pectin in apples attaches to carcinogenic material in the colon and escorts it from the body. Eating just one apple of any variety per day can help to minimize cancer-promoting substances in the body.

- *Garlic:* Cloves of garlic must be crushed or chopped to activate the chemical in garlic, called allicin, that is thought to slow tumor growth. Eating six to ten cloves of garlic per day packs a wallop of allicin, enough to reap its preventive benefits.

- *Onions:* Concentrated substances that contain sulphur and can turn off cell changes that lead to cancer growth are found in onions. Just one-half cup of onions per day, raw or cooked, may boost your cancer-prevention quotient.

- *Fiber:* Fiber speeds the flow of carcinogenic substances through the intestine, preventing the body's exposure to them for long periods of time. Soluble fiber is found in fruits and vegetables, while insoluble fiber is contained in whole grains. Experts recommend a combination of both kinds of fiber, which is particularly effective in preventing colon cancer and may be useful in preventing other cancers as well.

- *Flax oils:* They protect against free-radical damage and boost the work of antioxidants.

Anticancer Diets

If you have cancer, you may want to investigate the many diets that advocate eating specific foods to heal cancer. Each of these diets seems to have produced cases of "miracle cures," and almost all—except possibly the macrobiotic diet—result in excellent nutrition that improves health and consequently promotes a feeling of well-being, especially for people who have previously eaten poorly. Remember to consult with your doctor before making any dietary changes if you are undertaking any treatment. Also, these dietary measures should not be a substitute for your regular medical care. Some of the most popular diets follow.

Gerson Therapy. This diet operates on the premise that cancer is created by environmental toxins that overload the immune system and the liver. A diet primarily consisting of juice made from saltless, fat-free, organically grown fresh fruits and vegetables and calves' liver is believed to release toxins from the body and restore liver efficiency, possibly even healing cancer and certainly minimizing its risk of developing.

Livingston-Wheeler Therapy. This therapy is based on the theory that a weakened immune system can fall prey to certain bacteria that are found in the human body and other animals and, when activated, cause cancer. A diet low in animal products and protein, fats, and cholesterol and high in fresh fruits and vegetables, legumes, and whole grains is a staple tool of this therapy. Large quantities of vitamin A–rich foods, as well as injections of vitamins A, C, E, B_6, and B_{12}, are emphasized. Vaccines are another component of this therapy.

Macrobiotics. This Eastern-based diet advocates balancing foods that contain yang (hot) and yin (cold) energies to maximize health. Food is restricted by several criteria. It must be native to the part of the country or world in which you live, and it must be in season. For example, a New York resident would not eat Florida oranges nor eat summer fruit in the winter. Dairy products and most animal products are also forbidden. Because its many restrictions, a macrobiotic diet can result in vitamin deficiencies. Nevertheless, some adherents claim this diet has cured their cancers.

Ten-Percent-Fat Therapy. This therapy operates under the premise that fat in the diet contributes either directly or indirectly to many diseases, including cancer and heart disease, and thus should be minimized. Considering that most Americans eat a daily diet containing 37 percent fat, this therapy certainly seems to be headed in the right direction for promoting health and minimizing the risk of developing disease.

PSYCHOTHERAPY

Having cancer can profoundly complicate our lives, affecting many areas and touching each of our relationships. It can promote both short- and long-term stressors from the rigors of treatment and the concerns about employment and family care that it raises. For each person, the road from cancer discovery to recovery will be marked with different milestones. A profoundly complicated web of issues, from the existential to the immediate day-to-day treatment, may arise. Working through such issues to arrive at a point of meaning in each person's life is a process that often takes time, introspection, and deep thought, a process for which psychotherapy can be helpful.

Individual psychotherapy may be helpful in (1) identifying the specific sources of stress that result when cancer enters a person's life and (2) learning to successfully cope with them. If you decide to see a psychotherapist, she or he will evaluate your problem by discussing with you feelings and concerns, then make a recommendation about whether therapy would be beneficial and how long treatment might last. Short-term treatment could involve weekly appointments for three to six months, while long-term psychotherapy sessions may involve one to three weekly sessions for several years.

Through its empowerment, a cancer-support group can also help alleviate the long-term sources of stress, increase feelings of well-being, and promote better self-care. Group therapy can be a valuable tool for cancer patients to explore ways to handle the emotional stresses of their lives and to ameliorate symptoms and/or the experience of symptoms. Having cancer can itself be an alienating experience, and group therapy provides a forum for those with cancer to share their concerns and to validate their experiences. Family members and close friends of cancer patients are sometimes unable to cope with their feelings and so may deny the truth. This can make life more difficult and even more alienating for the cancer patient. A support group gives the cancer patient a whole world in which to share feelings and commonality.

Group therapy may have more power to heal than previously thought. Results of a related and much-touted study conducted at the Stanford University Medical School showed women with metastatic breast cancer participating in a breast-cancer support group lived twice as long as women who did not participate. Social isolation and alienation can cause chronic stress, which has been shown to have harmful effects on the body and can increase susceptibility to illness. Stress causes the body to release adrenal hormones that can suppress the immune system to some degree, making us more vulnerable to disease and allowing disease like cancer to progress more quickly.

Social support is also helpful because it increases our self-esteem, which may in turn increase self-care, thus improving our prognosis. So there are several clinical reasons to participate in group therapy besides the more obvious nurturing benefits.

If you decide to see a psychotherapist, ask him or her about his or her background and training, and the type of psychotherapy practiced. Some psychotherapists strictly follow one type of therapy, while others are eclectic and employ a variety of therapeutic techniques. (For more information about forms of therapy, see Chapter Two.)

Psychotherapy can be used with virtually any other alternative therapy, and when combined with mind-body therapies like biofeedback (Chapter Two), breathing for relaxation, hatha-yoga, hypnosis, and meditation, can produce powerful results. Besides promoting relaxation, the latter therapies can heighten personal insight.

CHAPTER NINE

Bone Health

Without the 206 bones in our body, we could not move nor keep our internal organs protected from damage. But many of us may be unaware that bones, just like muscles, are dependent on physical activity to maintain their strength and durability. We can observe the effect that exercise has on bone if we perform the same activity, tennis, for example, over and over. Because we use the forearm repeatedly to swing the racket, the bone in our forearm will increase in size and density. Of course, the opposite is also true. When we remain inactive for long periods of time and physical activity does not pull and stress the bones, our bodies lose bone mass, an effect seen in astronauts who experience weightlessness in space.

Thus, keeping bones healthy and strong with regular exercise is essential for maintaining everyone's health, both men and women. But maintaining bone mass is crucial for women, who are prone to losing substantial amounts of bone for much of their lives, beginning in their mid thirties. Women are also susceptible to a disease called osteoporosis, which weakens the bones so that they are prone to fracture or compression. Osteoporosis can begin as early as in a woman's twenties, but it is often not evident until the senior years. Another disease prevalent among women is called osteoarthritis. Osteoarthritis can strike at an early age like osteoporosis, but, again, it is common during the retirement years. It causes the cartilage in the joints to wear down, leading to pain and stiffness. We will discuss osteoporosis and osteoarthritis below, but first let us look at the natural processes that affect the bones—their health is essential in maintaining the health of the rest of the body, including the joints.

While our bones are hard on the surface, they're very porous inside. There are three types of bone in our body: long bones, found in the arms and legs, short bones, called vertebrae, located in the spine, and sesamoid bones, situated in the kneecaps. Bone tissue is made up of tiny particles of calcium and phosphorous in a honeycomb of protein-rich fibers called collagen. The calcium gives strength and hardness, and the collagen gives flexibility. Bones also contain fluoride, sodium, potassium, magnesium, citrate, and other trace elements to hold the calcium and phosphorus building blocks together.

You may be surprised to learn that blood vessels and nerves travel through the bone tissue just as they do the rest of the body. While 99 percent of calcium is used in bones, 1 percent is transported through the blood for vital functions like heart and other muscle contractions, blood clotting, and brain activities. Because of this blood flow, a constant exchange of calcium can take place between the bones and the rest of the body. If there is enough calcium traveling in the blood, particles of the mineral are taken in by the bone. However, if not enough calcium is in the blood to carry out other vital functions, some of the mineral leaves the bone and enters the bloodstream. This constant fluctuation in calcium accounts for our ever-changing bone mass—our bodies replace approximately 10 to 15 percent of our bone mass each year, and the average life of bone tissue in adults is ten years.

To build bone mass, the body needs many nutrients, including adequate levels of calcium, magnesium, phosphorus, vitamins A, C, D, and E, and trace minerals. Vitamin D may play the biggest role—without it, calcium cannot be absorbed by the body. By the time a woman is in her third decade, she has accumulated the bone mass for the rest of her life. The hormone estrogen plays an important role in accumulating bone mass by increasing calcium uptake by the body and by minimizing calcium loss from the bone. Following menopause, when estrogen stores have dwindled, the rate of bone loss accelerates for five to seven years, then stabilizes, but bone loss continues for the rest of a woman's life. Bone loss is also increased during the postmenopausal years because the body becomes more susceptible to actions of the parathyroid hormone, which also promotes calcium removal from the bones.

A common disease, osteoporosis can compound bone loss even further, during which bones can weaken and become fragile so that they may fracture or compress. Osteoporosis affects some 25 million Americans, mostly women, and may begin as early as in a woman's twenties by gradually siphoning bone mass from her body. Unfortunately, osteoporosis may not be discovered until it has progressed to the point of causing fractures in the postmenopausal years, when it is said to affect one in four women. In osteoporosis, the bones become weaker because the hard outer surface becomes thinner and the material inside more porous. Affected women may lose from one to eight inches in height as the bones, especially the spine, compress. In serious cases, the skeletal structure of the body can be completely altered. An outward curve of the upper spine can result, and the lower spine can curve inward. Shifts in skeletal structure can result in other changes in the body, including increased pressure on the nerves, pulled muscles, and joint stress that may lead to osteoarthritis.

Osteoarthritis, which affects 17 million Americans, mostly women in the middle years, affects the joints. This disease results in irregular growth and deterioration of the joint tissue called cartilage, which causes friction, irritation, and pain. To some degrees, osteoarthritis is common in every person over about 60 years of age, but only some —ten times more women than men—have symptoms of pain and discomfort. Joints can begin to deteriorate when the smooth cartilage, normally a buffer during joint movement, softens and becomes indented and frayed. It begins to lose its elasticity and becomes more easily damaged by movement. Eventually, large pieces of the cartilage can wear away, leaving parts of the bones exposed. In addition, small, irregular growths of cartilage and bone can develop in the joints, further exacerbating symptoms.

The symptoms of osteoarthritis differ from one person to another, but may include pain and stiffness in the joints of the body, and stiffness in the muscles surrounding the joint, which can weaken or contract unnaturally. Joint pain can become worse during cold and damp weather and upon waking, because stiffness can result from inactivity. Osteoarthritis in the spine can cause pressure on nerves, which can cause pain in the arms or legs, for example. Osteoarthritis usually affects only a few joints, and is more common in those that bear our weight because of the added stress. Thus, it will affect the hips, spine, knees, and feet before it occurs in the remaining joints, although the fingers and toes are commonly affected. The finger joints closest to the fingertips, the joint at the base of the thumb, and the joint at the base of the big toe are typical trouble spots. The finger joints are also vulnerable to the development of small bony growths called nodes. Osteoarthritis commonly occurs in the vertebrae of the lower spine (lumbar) and upper spine (cervical), but not in the joints of the wrists, elbows, and ankles.

Scientists are not sure what causes bone diseases like osteoarthritis and osteoporosis, but they know that genetic factors play a role. The risk factors for osteoporosis include being fair-skinned, very thin, anorexic, eating a low-calcium, very low-protein or very high-protein "meat-based" diet, consuming large amounts of alcohol, smoking, and being sedentary. But other risks can predispose women to getting osteoporosis as well. Those at higher risk include women of British, Northern European, Chinese, or Japanese ancestry; those with an immediate relative with the disease, and those who experienced early menopause—the earlier, the higher the risk. Also at greater risk are thin women of short or medium height (the bones of heavy and tall women become stronger to support their weight) and women with rheumatoid arthritis and endocrine disorders like diabetes. Mediterranean, and especially African-American, women are at low risk for the disease.

Women who are at risk for osteoporosis should watch for early signs of the disease. Although osteoporosis can affect any of your bones, it usually shows up first in the bones of the forearms and spine. However, loss of bone mass does not readily show up in X rays, because the hard, cortical outer bone can conceal a shrinking inner mass. Thus, a CAT scan (computerized axial tomography), which reveals bone density, should be performed.

There are other tests that you can request, including blood and urine samples, which indicate whether a large amount of calcium is being discharged from the bone or the body. Your diet, the use of laxatives, individual body metabolism, and the existence of other bone diseases can all affect calcium levels and, consequently, your test results.

An early indication that bones may be thinning can be found on the skin. If the skin on the back of your hand is loose and lacks pigment so that you can see the tiny veins, you may be deficient in collagen, the matrix found in the bones. Thin skin can also mean that you have rheumatoid arthritis, however, so be sure to have your condition diagnosed. Gum disease, an indication that calcium levels in the teeth are low, may be a sign of osteoporosis, although it may simply indicate poor dental hygiene.

Despite its prevalence, the cause of osteoarthritis remains a mystery to scientists. As is the case with many diseases, genetic factors are believed to set a predisposition for osteoarthritis, especially for the nodal variety affecting the fingers, but the rest of the picture remains unclear. Defective cartilage or defective joints, undetectable until disease occurs, may contribute to the development of osteoarthritis. Improper care of joints may also affect the joints. By not allowing an injured joint to heal properly before resuming activity, for example, or by overusing certain joints, we can increase our risk of developing osteoarthritis. Baseball players often develop the disease in the shoulder and elbow joints, while dancers are prone to osteoarthritic joints of the foot and ankle—in both cases, sites that are not typically affected by osteoarthritis. However, a majority of cases develop without indications of abuse, overuse, or defect, and it is those occurrences of osteoarthritis that scientists continue to probe.

Managing these diseases involves a combination of good nutrition, exercise, and an overall healthy lifestyle. Women who are predisposed to bone and joint diseases or who already have them may be somewhat frustrated with the allopathic approach—until recently it was assumed that osteoporosis and osteoarthritis were a natural part of the aging process. With current awareness that bone loss can be prevented with early intervention, allopathic treatment generally involves calcium supplements and a recommendation for increased exercise. But while supplements may be effective in increasing your calcium intake, it is your physical, emotional, and psychological disposition in conjunction with your other treatment that will help to enable you to prevent the disease through self-care. Standard osteoarthritis treatment can be somewhat disappointing. If aspirin tablets are not effective in relieving pain, drugs like corticosteroids may be used, which have the same harmful effects as the adrenal hormones released by the body during stress. The use of corticosteroids, furthermore, places you at risk for many other diseases—including osteoporosis.

Bone and joint diseases are *not* a losing battle. Bone loss can be stopped and osteoarthritis prevented from taking over our lives. Given the fundamental tools for prevention—good nutrition, exercise, emotional support, and a feeling of well-being—our bodies will do the rest. Learning how to incorporate natural therapies into our lives and how to manage our lives in a new and healthier context are the purposes *and* the approach of the natural therapies listed below.

BREATHING FOR RELAXATION (FOR OSTEOPOROSIS)

Relaxation is particularly important in maintaining bone health because the hormones released during the body's physiological reaction to stress, called the "fight or flight" response, affect the body's calcium levels in several ways. During stress, the adrenal glands release hormones that fire off increases in heart rate, metabolism, blood pressure, breathing rate, and muscle tension. Under the influence of adrenal hormones, increased amounts of calcium are depleted from the bone, and larger amounts of calcium are discharged in the urine. This hormonal release in the body may also decrease the amount of calcium absorbed by the intestines from food. Adrenal hormones affect vitamins that play a role in bone health as well. In their presence, levels of vitamin C are depleted, which are necessary for the production of the bone's connective tissue, collagen. In addition, if excess levels of vitamin D are present, adrenal hormones can accelerate the vitamin's destructive effect of decreasing calcium stores. If secretion of the adrenal hormones is constant, the normal alkaline base of the blood is altered, becoming acidic. To counteract this effect, vital calcium is released from the bones and discharged into the blood stream, restoring its alkalinity.

Since stress is by far the greatest promoter of blood acidity—coffee and alcohol also have this effect—the best natural defense against osteoporosis is to minimize the stress response. A change in breathing quality is one of the first and the most obvious signs that the body is launching a stress response. By interrupting this rapid-breathing response, we can slow or even avert the stress response and those harmful metabolic changes that accompany it. For details on how to breathe healthfully, see the belly-breathing practice in "Breathing for Relaxation," Chapter Three.

CHIROPRACTIC (FOR OSTEOPOROSIS)

The natural therapy of chiropractic advocates maintenance of the body's skeletal structure, primarily the spine, to protect and restore health. Disease or discomfort can result when any number of factors cause the spinal joints, which protect nerves in the spinal cord, to be locked out of place, upsetting the balance in the body. Misalignment can also reduce blood flow, cause pain and discomfort, and affect an array of other body functions, from the physiological to the emotional.

Chiropractic adjustments can slow the progression of both osteoporosis and osteoarthritis. During osteoporosis, the bones can shift out of alignment. The body responds by attempting to fuse the joints so that they can't move out of place. To do this, the body must tap into the calcium supply of the bones to lay down additional amounts at the joints. Besides accelerating osteoporosis, these calcium deposits can irritate osteoarthritic joints and intensify pain. Thus, a spinal realignment may be very helpful in slowing the progress of early stages of osteoporosis. It is not generally recommended for advanced stages of the disease when bones have become brittle, however.

Although chiropractic is an excellent form of therapy for musculoskeletal conditions like osteoporosis, there are several types of disorders for which it is inappropriate, including bone infection and cancer. In addition, if you have atherosclerosis or other problems with the arteries, manipulation of the neck and lower back should be avoided.

There are many other natural healing therapies that complement chiropractic treatment, including acupuncture, hatha-yoga, herbs, massage, meditation, and psychotherapy.

EXERCISE (FOR OSTEOPOROSIS)

Tall women are less prone to develop osteoporosis because their muscles and bones have become strong while carrying their body weight. The same principle applies to exercising for preventing osteoporosis. Any activity that pulls and stresses the long bones of the body can be a helpful ally against osteoporosis. While exercise can increase bone density and mass, the reverse is also true. By *not* performing any activity, we *lose* bone mass. Astronauts who experience weightlessness in space and people who are bedridden typically lose bone mass.

Thus, full-body activities like walking, cycling, or running are highly recommended for keeping our skeleton in good working order. And since weight-bearing bones are most affected by osteoporosis, any exercise that strengthens them—from walking to cycling to weight-lifting—can provide remarkable preventive benefits. Exercise also improves circulation, increases our energy level and prevents other disease as well. Aerobic exercise supplies a natural form of pain relief.

Activity that is too strenuous, of course, can have harmful effects, so don't begin a rigorous exercise program tomorrow—it could lead to injury! Begin slowly and gently, and increase the level of activity incrementally as your body becomes stronger. If you have osteoporosis, you should consult an exercise physiologist before beginning an exercise program. Your physiologist may recommend moderate exercise of slow movements without much strain or pounding, like hatha-yoga.

Aerobic Exercise

A safe and easy remedy, aerobic exercise involves working the major muscle groups of the body at least four times each week for at least twenty minutes, but preferably for forty minutes. Besides increasing bone mass, aerobic exercise has many other preventive benefits as well. It lowers risk of heart disease by decreasing blood pressure and increasing the "good" HDL cholesterol that prevents the "bad" LDL cholesterol from clogging the arteries. Aerobic exercise also improves circulation and, in addition to that, causes the body to release its natural painkilling endorphins and enkephalins.

To learn how to establish a walking or running regimen, see "Aerobic Exercise," Chapter Three.

Osteoporosis Bone Watch

In addition to performing exercises that strengthen your entire skeleton, a routine to tone and strengthen bones that are especially vulnerable to fracture, those that are largely made of porous bone—the hips, spine, and forearms—is recommended.

The following exercises can improve hip and forearm strength. Practice them daily to achieve the maximum benefit. (For exercises to strengthen the spine, see the following section on "Hatha-Yoga.")

Hip Kicks. Lie on your left side with your body straight and your head lying on your left arm, which is extended over your head. On the count of four, gently lift your right leg from the hip, raising it several inches from the left leg. Be sure that your foot is facing forward. Lower your leg on a count of four. Do this ten times to a count of two or until you tire. Now repeat the exercise, but flex your foot, that is, push the heel down and the toe up so that the foot is perpendicular to the leg. Do this ten times to a count of two, or until you feel discomfort. Turn on to your right side and repeat the series of exercises with your left leg. This exercise will cause some achiness at first, but within three days, the achiness will stop. Within a week, you will be able to increase your workout. Aim to ultimately perform two sets of fifty kicks with each leg.

Scissors Kicks. This is a more advanced exercise that you will be able to do after practicing stomach situps (see "Yoga," Chapter Seven) and hip kicks for several weeks. Lie flat on your back. Slowly raise legs straight into the air so that they are perpendicular to the floor and several inches apart. To a count of four, gently open legs about one and one-half feet apart. Be sure to keep your lower back pressed closely to the floor. Hold for a count of two. Bring the legs back together to a count of four. Repeat this several times. Now *slowly* open the legs as far as you can and hold for a count of two. Gradually close them again. Repeat this several times. Over time, increase scissor kicks to twenty-five.

Weight-Lifting

Wearing increased weight can increase muscle and bone mass in smaller bones like the wrist that normally don't bear much weight. You can buy a set of two-pound weights with cushioning that slips over the wrists or ankles. Wear them intermittently until you adjust to the extra weight, then during your whole exercise routine. To increase the strength of the wrists, incorporate the exercise below into your daily regimen.

Wrists.   Wearing wrist weights or, if you have osteoporosis, holding a soup can in your palm, lay your forearm on a flat surface with your palm facing up. Bend your wrist slowly upward as far as you can go. Hold for a count of two. Relax your wrist. Now repeat the exercise five to ten times, pausing for a moment if the muscle aches. Rest your wrist. Now turn your arm to the other side so that your wrist is dangling over the edge of the surface. Lift your wrist up as far as is comfortable. Hold for a count of two. Relax your wrist. Now repeat the exercise five to ten times, pausing for a moment if the muscle aches. Repeat the exercise using the other wrist.

HATHA-YOGA (FOR OSTEOPOROSIS)

In maintaining bone health, regular yoga practice can increase skeletal flexibility and gently strengthen muscles, which can lead to strong bones. Strong muscles are instrumental in preserving good posture and preventing structural-related diseases and skeletal malformations. Strong abdominal muscles can also take most of the workload off of the spine, thus reducing the possibility of injury and often eliminating lower back ache.

Hatha-yoga can also help relieve some of the specific symptoms related to osteoporosis. Women with this disease may experience a chronic ache along the spine or pain from a muscle spasm in the back muscles. When the muscles of the back must take an increased share of the load to support the upper half of the body if the spine has partially collapsed, they become overworked, tense, and achy. Mild yoga stretches can relieve these muscle spasms and stretch the spine ever so gently.

Yoga treatment involves practicing asanas (positions) throughout the month. (See Chapter Three for the following exercises.) For maximum effectiveness, first perform the belly-breathing practice (see "Breathing for Relaxation") and the practice meditation (see "Meditation"), then warm up with the sun salutation (see "Hatha-Yoga").

Yoga is safe and effective and can also be used in conjunction with any other natural therapy. Some positions may exacerbate conditions like hypertension or hernia, however. Be sure to take note of any precautions listed below.

The following asanas can be helpful for increasing skeletal flexibility and strengthening and stretching the muscles. Unless otherwise noted, most stretches should be held for only ten seconds initially. Gradually increase to two or even several minutes if it is comfortable.

Cobra. Lie on your stomach, and, bending your arms at the elbow, place your palms flat on the floor next to your chest. By putting weight on your hands and arms, slowly lift the chin. Hold the position for fifteen seconds. Now lift your chest from the floor, keeping your chin up. Hold that position for fifteen seconds. Slowly raise your torso from the floor and hold for thirty seconds, or as long as possible. When your flexibility improves, gradually increase this pose to two to three minutes.

Precautions: Do not perform this asana if you have hypertension or a hernia.

Child's Pose.   See "Hatha-Yoga," Chapter Four.

Single-Leg Lifts.   See "Hatha-Yoga," Chapter Seven.

Yoga Situp.   See "Hatha-Yoga," Chapter Seven.

Abdominal Rock.   See "Hatha-Yoga," Chapter Seven.

Free Pose.   See "Hatha-Yoga," Chapter Seven.

HOMEOPATHY (FOR OSTEOPOROSIS)

Homeopathy's gentle approach may be helpful in relieving some of the symptoms of osteoporosis by strengthening the body's defense against disease. Having osteoporosis can create chronic stress, which can have an adverse effect on our immune system. Taking homeopathic remedies can help to reactivate the body's immune system with substances that produce a similar set of symptoms in a healthy person. They can restore the body's own healing action and can relieve some of the symptoms of disease. Homeopathy provides a way for us to rebalance ourselves and makes us better able to manage our illness and the effects it creates in our lives.

If you are treating yourself, it's important to match your feelings and physical symptoms as closely as possible with the remedies listed below, just as a homeopath would. Unless otherwise noted, take a dose of 30c daily. *Stop* taking medication once discomfort or other symptoms begin to diminish. If your medication has no effect, it usually indicates that you have taken the wrong remedy. In that case, review your symptoms and, being as specific as possible, match them to another remedy. You should also consult with an appropriate health professional before taking any remedy.

Homeopathy may be used in conjunction with some therapies like acupuncture (Chapter Four), chiropractic and hypnosis (Chapter Eight), or psychotherapy (Chapter Two). But it should generally not be used simultaneously with aromatherapy or herbs because the former's essential oils may inactivate the homeopathic solution, as will coffee, alcohol, tobacco, perfumed cosmetics, and pungent household cleansers.

- *Phosphorus:* This remedy can provide relief for shooting pains from the joints or bones, and it will tend to counteract bone fragility and weakness and thus help prevent fractures in the spine and other joints. It is especially effective for maladies that worsen during weather changes and on humid and warm days and improve with cold weather.

- *Ruta graveolens:* If you feel pain and achiness in the bones, especially in the spinal column and the limbs, and symptoms are worse during cold weather and when you're lying flat, this will often have a beneficial effect.

- *Arsenicum album:* If limbs, hands, and feet are weighing you down, your back is painful, and symptoms exacerbate late at night and improve with heat, taking a dose of this can help your symptoms.

IMAGERY (FOR OSTEOPOROSIS)

Relaxation imagery helps to relieve stress, which is known to contribute to calcium loss from the bones and can exacerbate osteoporosis. Thus, alleviating feelings of anxiety through imagery can be helpful in combating and preventing the disease. Try the relaxation imagery technique (see "Imagery," Chapter Three) twice daily to relax. If you suffer from osteoporosis, you may want to adapt the exercise to include some very strong images. For example, develop a scene in which your bones open up and let more calcium march in, building a steadfast fortress to keep the passage open for new calcium troops. Don't forget to make the images vivid so that your mind will be convinced of their authenticity!

Imagery can be used in conjunction with any natural therapy but offers its greatest advantages when combined with biofeedback (Chapter Two), hypnosis (Chapter Eight), and other relaxation techniques.

MASSAGE (FOR OSTEOPOROSIS)

Many women with osteoporosis learn that they have a fractured vertebrae when they have not ever felt pain. Usually, however, there is pain—either a chronic ache along the spine or pain from a muscle spasm in the back muscles. Because the muscles of the back must take an increased share of the load to support the upper half of the body if the spine has partially collapsed, muscle spasm and ache can result. Massage is very effective at releasing muscle spasms and can increase the flow of blood to your back. It can also release emotional tension that may have lodged in the muscles.

The massage warmup will loosen tissue (see "Massage," Chapter Three). Then ask your helper to apply the specific application below.

Massage can be used in conjunction with any alternative therapy, and is often combined with acupressure, aromatherapy, and chiropractic.

Precautions: Do not massage areas of varicose veins.

To Relieve Backaches and/or Muscle Spasms

First, apply long, gliding strokes to the whole back, beginning with the buttocks and working up to the top. Then, with the palm of your hand, rub six-inch circles in a counterclockwise direction on the buttocks, then to the lower back, then to the rest of the back. You're ready to release tension from the deep muscles. Start with the buttocks, taking large amounts of skin and muscle into your hands and working them by squeezing, kneading, and rolling. Work your way up the back. You'll feel the tissue soften and become more pliable as you release tensions. Finish by lightly brushing the entire back with your fingertips.

MEDITATION (FOR OSTEOPOROSIS)

During osteoporosis, meditation can provide an outlet for gaining peace of mind. Meditation is a quiet state of existence in which our thoughts do not distract us. Thus, concerns about health that may cause anxiety can be minimized by practicing meditation regularly. The resulting relaxation is also helpful in minimizing discomforts that can be heightened by anxiety. Another benefit, the deep relaxation promoted during meditation, is helpful in maintaining calcium levels in the body. Stress causes release of the adrenal hormones that increase the use of calcium by the body. Try the practice meditation (see "Meditation," Chapter Three) twice daily to relax. If you are experiencing achiness, try to observe anxious thoughts that accompany pain and let go of them.

Meditation can be combined with virtually any natural therapy.

NUTRITIONAL THERAPY
(FOR OSTEOPOROSIS)

Maintaining calcium levels in the body is a challenge for most women. First of all, most women only take in about 500 to 600 milligrams of calcium each day—about half of what they need to satisfy the body's needs. Second, it's hard to keep our sights set on eating nonfat yogurt when calcium levels in the body are affected by everything from stress to alcohol to laxatives—everything under the sun, including, yes, sunshine. For all of the trouble, is calcium really worth it?

Let's find out. For proper bone formation and development, the body needs many nutrients, including vitamins A, C, D, and small amounts of minerals, including phosphorus and fluoride. But vitamin D may be the most important component in the bone process next to calcium—it prepares calcium for use by the body, and without it, we couldn't use calcium. The best source of vitamin D is made by the body when exposed to sunlight. Between fifteen minutes and one hour of sunlight per day, depending on the shade of your skin (fair-skinned people need less), can provide the body with enough of the ultraviolet (UV) rays to synthesize valuable vitamin D. Because UV rays cannot penetrate window glass, you must be outside for your body to absorb them. Protect your eyes, though, because constant exposure to UV light can damage them and cause cataracts.

Too much vitamin D can have just the opposite effect of helping your body receive calcium; it causes large amounts of calcium to be taken from the bones. If we obtain vitamin D from UV rays, the body has a natural mechanism that turns off its synthesis when stores are adequate. If your source is food or vitamin supplements, however, excessive levels of vitamin D are stored in the body fat and liver. Slower metabolism during the middle years can further affect calcium synthesis because the liver and kidneys do not work as efficiently to utilize the stored vitamin D.

Other vitamins are needed by the body for proper bone development. Vitamin A is necessary to help the bones grow their correct length. Vitamin C is used in the formation of collagen-forming connective tissue, and also aids in healing bone fractures. Vitamin C is water-soluble and excess amounts are discharged through the urine within an hour after consumption, so it's important to eat vitamin-C rich foods on a daily basis. Fortunately, the food sources for vitamin C are widespread and popular. However, some factors interfere with vitamin C absorption, including the use of birth control pills and overuse of laxatives.

As mentioned, there are many factors that can inhibit calcium absorption, perhaps one good reason why calcium deficiency is so widespread. The use of laxatives and a very high-fiber diet can interfere with nutrient absorption because food passes too quickly through the intestinal tract for nutrients to be extracted. Bran fiber, in particular, increases the loss of calcium, as well as of phosphorus, magnesium, iron, and zinc. Other nutrients that interfere with calcium absorption are called phytates, found in wheat and oat bran, and oxalates, which naturally occur in some green, leafy vegetables including spinach, beet greens, Swiss chard, and rhubarb. Meat, sodas, brewer's yeast (used to make beer), and processed foods all contain phosphorus, high levels of which reduce calcium intake by the body. Most minerals are interdependent—that is, an imbalance in one mineral usually results in an imbalance in another mineral. The calcium-to-phosphorus ratio is 1:1, or better yet, 2:1, and if calcium is exceeded by phosphorus, the result can be a calcium deficiency. So when we indulge in many foods that are high in phosphorus, we are, in effect, reducing our calcium stores.

Other factors that can impede calcium levels in the body include a high-fat, high-sugar, low-protein or high-protein diet, large amounts of alcohol, coffee (four or more cups per day), fasting or crash dieting, megavitamin supplements of vitamin A, and drugs—tetracycline, corticosteroids, anticonvulsants, antacids containing aluminum, diuretics, and thyroid supplements. Coffee, alcohol, and smoking all increase calcium usage by altering the blood's alkaline base to become acidic. Calcium is released to restore the blood's alkalinity.

But all is not lost. There are effective ways to maximize intake of calcium, the body's most important mineral. After all, without it, we couldn't even move, play sports, or go to the refrigerator to get nonfat yogurt. The best way to promote healthy bones is to maintain adequate levels of calcium and other needed nutrients through nutritional sources. Nonfat dairy products like yogurt are a good source because they contain proportionately high amounts of the mineral. However, dairy products are also high in cholesterol, and a diet high in dairy products increases constipation. In addition, milk contains substances that inhibit calcium absorption. Try some vegetarian sources of calcium such as kale, watercress, parsley, mustard and collard greens, broccoli and alfalfa sprouts. For a list of foods containing good sources of calcium, and the vitamins needed for calcium synthesis, see "Nutritional Therapy," Chapter Three. Instead of using laxatives frequently, get more exercise, drink more liquids, and eat more fresh vegetables and fruits. Finally, you may want to take a calcium supplement. Listed below are the daily levels of calcium recommended by most experts for different stages of our lives.

MILLIGRAMS OF CALCIUM PER DAY

Children	
Birth–1 year	360
1–10 years	540
11–18	1,200
Premenopausal women	1,000
Estrogen-treated women	1,000
Postmenopausal women	1,500
Pregnant or nursing women	
under 19 years	2,000
over 19 years	1,400

Vitamin Supplements

Calcium. Since most of us don't consume nearly the amount of calcium we need for a healthy future, mineral supplements are a viable option. Most nutrition experts agree that an intake of 2,000 milligrams of calcium daily from both diet and supplements can be tolerated without any adverse effects. Unclear is whether high amounts of supplements alone are tolerated. Excessive levels of calcium can cause arteriosclerosis, hardening of the arteries from calcification, and "kidney stones" (mineral deposits in the kidney). If you choose to take a supplement, be sure to take one with adequate levels of the mineral. Calcium levels in some of the more popular supplements are listed below.

PERCENT OF CALCIUM

Calcium carbonate	40
Calcium lactate	13
Calcium gluconate	9

Avoid bonemeal and dolomite—although high in calcium, they both tend to contain substantial amounts of lead and other toxic metals that remain permanently stored in the body. Antacid supplements that contain only calcium are a great source, but, as previously mentioned, avoid those containing aluminum—they will have the opposite effect.

When you take calcium supplements, drink a full glass of water. In order for them to be absorbed by the body, sufficient hydrochloric acid is necessary. Thus, calcium supplements should be taken on an empty stomach unless your stomach does not produce much acid, a common condition among elderly people. In this case, supplements should be taken with meals. Very high-dosage calcium supplements may reduce the absorption of other important minerals such as manganese, zinc, and iron.

Precautions: Levels of calcium intake greater than those recommended can result in mineral deposits in the kidneys ("kidney stones"). People with kidney stones should take calcium supplements only under the supervision of a physician.

Vitamin D. If dietary sources are scarce, or you live in a cold climate and are always bundled up so the UV rays cannot penetrate the skin, you may want to take a vitamin D supplement of 5 milligrams, the U.S. recommended daily dietary allowance. An additional 5 milligrams is recommended if you are pregnant or breastfeeding. Because vitamin D is fat-soluble, however, excess amounts are stored in the liver and body fat, and very high amounts can have toxic effects.

Vitamin A. The recommended daily dietary allowance of vitamin A is 800 RE (one RE = 1 microgram of retinol or 6 micrograms of beta-carotene). Amounts much more than that can have the opposite effect by triggering bone loss. Because vitamin A is fat-soluble, excess amounts are stored in the liver and body fat, and very high amounts can have toxic effects.

Vitamin C. The recommended daily allowance of vitamin C is 60 milligrams, found in one medium-sized orange. However, stress, coffee, and alcohol, among other factors, can reduce vitamin C stores. Megavitamin supplements in the amount of 250 to 1,000 milligrams are what is usually available, but if you cannot find smaller quantities, you can break the larger-dosage vitamins up. Excess vitamin C is discharged from the body in less than an hour, so it won't cause harmful effects, but splitting up your dosage —half in the morning and half at night—may increase absorption.

See "Nutritional Therapy," Chapter Three, for foods containing good dietary sources of vitamins and minerals needed for proper bone development.

ACUPRESSURE
(FOR OSTEOARTHRITIS)

As with any Western medical diagnosis, osteoarthritis has many possible causes in Chinese medicine. It may result from deficiency of the kidneys, the root of the body's energy. It can also result from deficiency of *jing*, or "essence," which is also associated with the kidneys. Another cause may be liver deficiency.

However, osteoarthritis may also result from excess *chi* stagnation, blood stagnation, or a condition known as *Wind-Damp-Bi*, a pattern where the qualities of "wind" and "damp" have settled into the meridians.

Each cause of arthritis has different symptoms. For example, "wind" arthritis becomes worse when the wind blows and during movement. "Heat" arthritis can be noted by inflammation and redness. When you touch these joints, you will feel the heat. In "cold" arthritis, joints are more painful when the temperature drops or other weather changes take place. "Damp" arthritis means joints are most irritated when humidity increases, and they will feel heavy at that time. Arthritis can be any one or a combination of these types. Eating foods that are cold, damp, or heat-producing can also contribute to the pain of arthritis.

Treatment involves expelling the wind, damp, cold, or heat from the body and treating other energy systems to balance *chi* and to move and nourish blood in the body. Acupressure treatment involves a variety of point-stimulation techniques that redirect the flow of energy in the body, and, in the process, prompt secretion of the body's painkilling chemicals. Acupuncture is based on the same principles as acupressure, but it must be performed by a skilled professional with years of training (for more information, see "Acupuncture," Chapter Three).

Described below are various acupressure remedies for osteoarthritis. Unless otherwise noted, you should press each acupressure point firmly but gently for two to three minutes, or until you feel relief. For further instructions on how to apply acupressure, see "Acupressure," Chapter Three.

While acupressure is a gentle, safe treatment when used properly, some precautions should be taken. You should never use acupressure as a *primary* treatment to relieve conditions you may have along with osteoarthritis, such as excessive bleeding, vaginal discharges, or undiagnosed pain, each of which can be an indication of serious illness requiring prompt medical care. Be sure to consult a physician.

For Finger Joints

- *TW 4:* Find this point in the hollow in middle of the wrist on the back of the hand.
- *Large intestine 10:* With the elbow flexed and the palm facing down, you can find this point two finger-widths below the elbow crease, pressing against the bone.
- *TW 5:* This point is located on the outside of the forearm, with the palm facing down, about three finger-widths above the wrist crease and halfway between the two bones.
- *Pericardium 7:* Find this point at the center of the crease in the middle of the wrist on the inside of the arm.

For Knees

- *Gallbladder 33:* Locate this point behind the joint where the knee is bent, in the depression on the outside of the external knee eye, between the tendon and the bone, or about four finger-widths above *gallbladder 34* (below).

- *Stomach 36:* This point is located on the calf, four finger-widths below the bottom of the kneecap, one finger-width outside the shinbone. The point is on a muscle, which you can feel move if you flex your foot.

For Hips (Local Points)

- *Gallbladder 31:* You can locate this point on the outside of the thigh about seven inches from the crease of the knee. When you stand with your hands at your sides, the point is where the end of the middle finger touches the thigh.

- *Bladder 30:* You'll find this point on the lower back at the level of the fourth sacral hole, one and one-half inches from the spine.

For Hips (Distal Points)

- *Gallbladder 34:* This point is situated on the outside of the leg just beneath the head of the fibula.

- *Gallbladder 40:* You'll find this point in the indentation in front of the outer anklebone.

For Shoulders (Local Points)

- *Large intestine 11:* When the elbow is flexed and the palm is facing down, this point is in the depression at the outer end of the elbow crease.

- *TW 14:* You'll find this point behind and below the shoulder joint, in the depression found about one inch behind *large intestine 15.* (See illustration at back of book.)

- *TW 15:* In the depression between the muscle and bone, at the end of the humerus where it meets the shoulder bone, you'll find this point. A hollow appears on the point when the arms is lifted. (See illustration at back of book.)

For Shoulders (Distal Points)

- *TW3:* This point is situated on the back of the hand in the hollow just between the fourth and fifth metacarpal bones.

- *Large intestine 10:* With the elbow flexed and the palm facing down, you can find this point two finger-widths below the elbow crease, pressing against the bone.

For Lower Spine

Hold the next two points simultaneously:

- *Small intestine 3:* This point is located on the outer side of the little finger, in the depression behind the base joint, when making a fist.

- *Bladder 62:* Find this point in the depression directly below the outer anklebone.

- *Bladder 23:* This point is located one and one-half inch from the center of the spine between the second and third lumbar vertebrae.

- *Bladder 40:* You'll find this point at the midpoint of the crease behind the knee.

CHIROPRACTIC
(FOR OSTEOARTHRITIS)

Preserving musculoskeletal health of the spine and nervous system is integral to preventing illness with the surgery-free, drug-free therapy of chiropractic. However, when the spinal joints, which protect nerves in the spinal cord, become locked out of place, they can upset the balance in the body. This misalignment can alter a wide range of body functions, causing effects from immediate discomfort to degenerative diseases.

Chiropractic is very effective in treating arthritic problems. Because chiropractic adjustments help to boost the body's enzymatic, metabolic, and nervous systems, the body is able to marshal resources to the areas of damage to restore them. In addition, soft-tissue manipulation stimulates the circulatory and lymph systems, which helps to clear the toxins from the joints, minimizing irritation. Soft-tissue manipulation also releases tension in the muscles surrounding the joints, increasing joint movement and rotation. Together, these techniques help to restore the body's homeostatic balance without the side effects of drugs. While drugs may reduce some of the painful symptoms of arthritis, they do nothing about treating the condition itself.

Although chiropractic is an excellent form of therapy for musculoskeletal conditions like osteoarthritis, there are several types of disorders for which it is inappropriate, including bone infection and cancer. In addition, if you have atherosclerosis or other problems with the arteries along with osteoarthritis, manipulation of the neck and lower back should be avoided.

There are many other natural healing therapies that complement chiropractic treatment, including acupuncture, aromatherapy, hatha-yoga, herbs, massage, meditation, and psychotherapy.

EXERCISE (FOR OSTEOARTHRITIS)

Striking a delicate balance between rest and exertion is the key to exercise therapy for those with osteoarthritis. Complete rest will stiffen the joints and overexertion will make them sore. Encouraged is a moderate amount of nonstrenous non-weight-bearing activities from yoga to swimming to range-of-motion exercises. Not only can these activities provide remarkable relief for those with osteoarthritis, they can improve circulation and overall health.

Exercises that increase the range of joint motion increase the amount of synovial fluid in the joints. This fluid bathes the cartilage and bone, thus minimizing pain. Too much exercise, however, can have just the opposite effect on the joints and increase pain. Such observations once led practitioners to overlook exercise, one of the most helpful osteoarthritis remedies, for fear of increasing joint pain. Bed rest was the common medical advice offered by physicians to those with osteoarthritis not so long ago.

Today, practitioners are well aware of the useful benefits of exercise, and many recommend a daily regimen of gentle stretching exercises (see "Hatha-Yoga") and range-of-motion exercises (see below), while swimming and walking may be alternated throughout the week. For information on how to begin a walking program, see "Aerobic Exercise," Chapter Three.

Range-of-Motion Exercises

Exercise is important to reestablish mobility and a complete range of motion, which osteoarthritis diminishes. The following range-of-motion exercises relieve stiffness and increase the amount of synovial fluid in the joints, which reduces pain. Practice them daily. If you cannot complete the full movement, go as far as you can, then gradually increase the range of motion.

Fingers.   Rest your hand and forearm on a flat surface. Slowly curl the ends of your fingers and thumb under (the last joint only). Hold for five seconds. Now make a tight fist. Hold for five seconds. Release your grip, and let the fingers lay flat on the surface for ten seconds. Stretch your hand open by extending fingers and thumb as far as possible for five seconds. Repeat with the other hand.

Wrists.   Lay your forearm on a flat surface with the wrist bent so that your hand is dangling over the edge. Now contract the muscles in the arm and hand so that your hand is level with your forearm. While keeping muscles taut, bend your wrist upward so that hand becomes perpendicular to the floor. Now, slowly, and with resistance, swing your wrist downward, so that hand is perpendicular to the floor. Practice two to three times daily.

Shoulders and Elbows.   Stand erect. Put your hands behind your head just above the neck while bending elbows out to the side. Contract muscles in your arms and bend at the shoulders to bring your elbows forward, almost to the front of your face, or as far as you can go. Now, while holding resistance in the muscles, with hands still resting on your head, push elbows as far back as you can. Keep your chin slightly raised. Repeat the exercise several times.

Shoulders. This exercise will increase the range of motion in the arms as well as enhance upper-body posture. Stand erect and extend your arms out to the sides. Lock your elbows and flex the hands so your palms are flat and perpendicular to the floor. Push with your arms as if you were trying to move something big. Make small backward circles with your arms, being sure to contract the muscles during movement. Do this fifty times, then rest. Then do fifty more and rest.

Hips. Lie on your back with legs spread apart several inches. Contract leg muscles while slowly spreading legs apart. First spread them apart about one foot. Hold for a count of four. Then expand them one more foot. Hold for a count of four. Now extend them as far apart as possible. Hold for a count of two. Slowly slide legs together. Now slowly slide legs apart as far as they can go. Hold for a count of two. Bring them back together. Extend them again as far as they can go, but hold for four. Bring them together.

Hips and Knees. Lie flat on the floor with legs about one and one-half feet apart. Slowly turn your knees and feet toward each other several inches, bending from the hip. Hold for a count of two. Bring feet to their original position. Turn them together again, but this time closer than the last time. Hold for a count of two. Relax them.

Ankles. Sit on a high chair so that feet are dangling above the floor. Flex the foot slightly so that toes are pointed upward and the heels are pointed downward. Hold for a count of two. Release the position, and let the feet dangle for a count of two. Flex the foot again, this time a little more pronounced. Hold for a count of two, then release. Turn the feet so that they're each facing outward, and repeat the exercise. Now turn the feet so that they're each facing each other and repeat the exercise.

HATHA-YOGA (FOR OSTEOARTHRITIS)

Yoga's slow movements and gentle pressures can be very helpful in relieving osteoarthritis by reaching deep into troubled joints. Asanas increase flexibility of the joints and gently stretch tight muscles around the joints, both targets of osteoarthritic pain. Hatha-yoga has some other preventive benefits as well. In general, standing asanas strengthen the muscles of the legs, buttocks, abdomen, back, and shoulders. Strong muscles are instrumental in preserving good posture and in preventing structural-related diseases and skeletal malformations.

Yoga treatment involves practicing asanas throughout the month. (See Chapter Three for the following exercises.) For maximum effectiveness, first perform the belly-breathing practice (see "Breathing for Relaxation") and the practice meditation (see "Meditation"), then warm up with the sun salutation (see "Hatha-Yoga").

The asanas listed below can be helpful for increasing skeletal flexibility and strengthening and stretching the muscles. Unless otherwise noted, most stretches should be held for only ten seconds initially. Gradually increase to two or even several minutes if it is comfortable. If you have severe osteoarthritis, limit your daily yoga routine to several five-minute sessions.

Yoga is safe and effective and can also be used in conjunction with any other natural therapy. Some positions may exacerbate conditions like hypertension or hernia, however. Be sure to take note of any precautions for each exercise listed below.

Neck Twist. Place your elbows on a flat surface with your arms bent and your hands near your face. Sit close enough to the table to place each of your palms on your ears, letting the weight of your head rest on your hands and arms. Gently drop your head forward slightly, until you can clasp your hands together behind the skull of your head. With your hands, push your head down slowly until your chin touches your chest, or as far as you can go. Hold this position for a count of four. Now, without moving your arms, turn your head very slowly and rest your chin against your left arm. With your right hand, clasp the back of the head. Turn the head slowly to the left as far as you can. Hold for a count of four. Now, without moving the arms, repeat the action on your right side. Relax the position by dropping your head on the table.

Knee Stretch. Sit on the floor with your back straight and your legs extended in front of you. Bend the knees and bring the legs and feet toward you. Grasp the feet and bring the soles of the feet together. Hold that position for a count of six, or as long as is comfortable. Now gently pull your feet in toward your body and simultaneously press your knees toward the floor. Hold for a count of six or as long as is comfortable. As your flexibility improves, you will be able to bring your knees closer and closer to the floor.

Leg Pull.   Sit with your legs extended straight before you. Your back should be straight. Clasp your hands on your legs just below your knees, rounding your back slightly. To a count of five, bend slightly forward, pulling your trunk toward your knees. Go as far as is comfortable, with the ultimate goal of coming about one foot above the knee.

Spinal Twist.   See "Hatha-Yoga," Chapter Four.

Cobra.   See "Hatha-Yoga (for Osteoporosis)," above.

HERBS (FOR OSTEOARTHRITIS)

Because herbs are adaptogenic, allowing the body to take whatever it needs from them and releasing the rest, they are wonderful for treating inflammatory conditions like arthritis. Herbs may be helpful in a number of ways. They can help to alleviate inflammation of the joints, can provide nutrients for rebuilding the joints, and may help to rebalance the body's immune system, which is often thrown off by arthritis, exacerbating joint irritation.

Taking the herbs below in the recommended quantities should produce some relief right away. Once symptoms begin to subside, stop taking the herb. Of course, the effects of some herbs that stimulate the immune system will not be evident right away. In all cases, do *not* take the herb for longer periods or in greater doses than recommended below. You should also consult with your health professional before undertaking any herbal treatment.

Herbs should not be taken while using aromatherapy or homeopathy, but can be combined with most other natural therapies.

For more information on healing herbs, see "Herbs," Chapter Three.

Vervain or Blue Vervain (*Verbena hastata*). An encyclopedic array of uses of this aspirinlike herb since the time of the ancient Egyptians, Greeks, and Romans to the present make its leaves, flowers, and roots cherished. A species of this is available in Europe, cousin to that available in the United States. An anti-inflammatory agent and pain reliever, this herb can be useful for relieving a variety of minor discomforts, from headache to aching joints. Vervain also has a mild laxative effect.

Precautions: Vervain may slow heart rate and restrict breathing in some people. Thus, anyone with a history of heart disease or a respiratory condition such as asthma should *avoid* vervain. Because vervain stimulates the uterus and the intestine, pregnant women and those with gastrointestinal disorders should *avoid* this herb. Do not give this herb to children. Elderly people should begin with low doses and gradually increase them.

Preparation: For an infusion, steep one and one-half teaspoons of herb in a cup of boiling water for fifteen minutes. Drink no more than four cups per day. In a tincture, use one teaspoon no more than three times per day.

Echinacea (*Echinacea angustifolia*). The roots of this plant, a member of same family as the dandelion, were once treasured by Native Americans. Echinacea was then discovered by Europeans, who use this herb for its ability to fortify the immune system to both prevent and fight infections. Echinacea may be helpful for those with osteoarthritis because it contains a chemical that helps to prevent reduction in the fluid that lubricates the joints. If you have arthritis, echinacea should only be used in consultation with your physician. For more information, see "Herbs," Chapter Eight.

Nettles (*Urtica dioica*). The leaves and stems of this old-time favorite have been popular since ancient times to reduce inflammation of the joints during arthritis and gout. While folk remedies use the warmth generated from the sting of the hairlike bristles found on the plant to soothe aching joints, most herbalists recommend, in addition, drinking an infusion to help boost the restorative process in the joints. Nettles also improve circulation to and from the joints. For more information, see "Herbs," Chapter Five.

Turmeric (*Curcuma longa*). The roots of this member of the same family as ginger are prized by those with arthritis for their ability to reduce pain and inflammation. But turmeric provides aid in another way by supplying valuable nutrients for rebuilding healthy joints. Turmeric also has an anticlotting ability, making it valuable in reducing heart-disease risk.

Precautions: Because of its anticlotting ability, turmeric should not be used by those with anticlotting disorders such as hemophilia. It should not be given to children or elderly people. Pregnant women should avoid it.

Preparation: For a decoction, steep one teaspoon of dried root in a cup of boiling water for fifteen to twenty minutes. Drink no more than three cups per day.

HEAT THERAPY
(FOR OSTEOARTHRITIS)

While joint pain often becomes aggravated by cold and dampness, heat and moisture are universally recognized for providing comfort and analgesia. The use of moisture makes heat therapy doubly effective because water carries the heat and intensifies its effect. For people with osteoarthritis, heat therapy can relieve pain and restore mobility to the joints.

The simplest way to apply a heat treatment is by using a hot-water bottle on the aching joints. Another is to take a hot bath—with or without Epsom salts—which not only relieves pain but promotes relaxation. But in addition, many types of heat therapy, from using sleeping bags to liniment compresses to paraffin "baths," can be used to alleviate pain and discomfort from osteoarthritis.

Sleeping Bag

Whether donning thermal underwear or zipping into a sleeping bag, you will find the cocoon effect is the same. A uniform warmth wraps around the body, keeping the joints warm and dry. Try this technique if your joints are particularly sensitive to cold and dampness.

Hot, Moist Compress

A hot, moist compress on the area around and including the joint can be very effective in relieving joint pain as well as relaxing the muscles around the joint. Saturate a towel with hot but not scalding water. Wring out excessive moisture and fold in half. Lie down and place the towel immediately over the area for about ten to fifteen minutes. To maximize effectiveness, keep a bowl of very hot water at your bedside to refresh the compress every five minutes. A variation on this technique, called a fomentation, utilizes a wool-blanket material to retain heat that is lined with a cotton material (a sheet, perhaps) to retain moisture. Follow the same instructions for a compress, but immerse the cotton in hot water. Then cover with the dry, wool material. Leave on for twenty to forty minutes. Protect the bony areas of the body by lifting the fomentation occasionally to allow steam to escape. For acutely painful joints, apply this technique two to three times each day.

Liniment Packs

Liniments, another common treatment for aching joints, are very effective because they create heat to relieve pain. A liniment utilizes one or a mixture of various chemicals applied on a cloth to a troubled area. Chemicals combine to generate heat when placed on your skin, and can relieve pain and restore mobility. The same effect is found in commercial heat rubs. Try using crushed mustard seeds or castor oil on a hot, damp cloth and applying to the troubled areas using the instructions above for a compress or fomentation.

Paraffin (Wax) "Baths"

A paraffin bath is a comforting technique that allows soothing heat to penetrate all of the nooks and crannies of your aching hand. A paraffin bath actually uses a type of wax that melts at lower temperatures than candle wax, and can be purchased at your local pharmacy. Melt it in a double boiler. Do not melt the pan directly on an electric or gas stove because the wax catches on fire easily. Let it cool until a thin film of wax begins to form on the surface. Then immerse each hand, one at a time, into the mixture and pull out quickly. Let the wax dry for a minute, then repeat several times. Ask a friend to wrap each hand in a towel or plastic wrap to retain the heat. Let the wax rejuvenate the joints for twenty to thirty minutes before removing.

HOMEOPATHY
(FOR OSTEOARTHRITIS)

Homeopathy may be very helpful in relieving osteoarthritis because it gently stimulates the body's immune system with substances that produce a similar set of symptoms in a healthy person. The gentle healing effects of homeopathy can help to restore balance in the immune system and minimize symptoms of osteoarthritis.

If you are treating yourself, it's important to match your feelings and physical symptoms as closely as possible with the remedies listed below, just as a homeopath would. Unless otherwise noted, take a dose of 30c daily. *Stop* taking medication once discomfort or other symptoms begin to diminish. You should consult with an appropriate health professional before taking any remedy.

Homeopathy may be used in conjunction with some therapies like acupuncture (Chapter Three), chiropractic and hypnosis (Chapter Eight), or psychotherapy (Chapter Two). But it should generally not be used simultaneously with aromatherapy or herbs because the former's essential oils may inactivate the homeopathic solution, as will coffee, alcohol, tobacco, perfumed cosmetics, and pungent household cleansers.

- *Rhus toxicodendron:* If the joints in your hands or feet are stiff in the morning, and feel better with gentle, continuous movement or heat, this is the remedy of choice.

- *Bryonia alba:* When joint pain is severe but improves with coolness and rest and worsens with heat or movement, you can often get relief from this remedy.

- *Pulsatilla:* If heat increases joint pain, and you feel somewhat moody or tearful, this remedy can make a difference.

- *Calcarea carbonica:* If joints feel cool, and changes in weather make the joints achy and stiff, try this remedy, which can often help.
- *Arnica montana:* When cold and dry weather causes severe pain in the joints, this remedy can bring great benefit.

IMAGERY (FOR OSTEOARTHRITIS)

Relaxation imagery may be helpful in relieving the discomforts of osteoarthritis. By envisioning comforting images, you can instill peace and tranquility in mind and body and subdue symptoms of pain. You may even help to counteract the progression of the disease by envisioning that it is being swept from your body. Try the relaxation imagery technique (see "Imagery," Chapter Three) twice daily to relax. To counteract the disease's progress, adapt the exercise to include images of your joints being bathed in a warm and soothing liquid that carries away toxins and deposits from whatever area ails you. If you are experiencing pain, envision a light and gentle breeze blowing into the joints and freeing them from discomfort.

Imagery can be used in conjunction with any natural therapy but offers its greatest advantages when combined with biofeedback (Chapter Two), hypnosis (Chapter Eight), and other relaxation techniques.

MASSAGE (FOR OSTEOARTHRITIS)

In osteoarthritis, the muscles tend to contract unnaturally as a result of joint stiffness. Emotional tension, perhaps caused by anxiety about the disease, can also lodge in the muscles. Massage techniques can reach deeply into troubled muscles and restore their suppleness. Massage therapy also stimulates the blood and lymph systems, promoting the removal of toxins that can accumulate in the joints.

Try the massage warmup to loosen tissue (see "Massage," Chapter Three) using peanut, olive, or castor oil. Then, to contact and release trouble spots, use the deep-muscle technique listed below for painful muscles. Ask your helper to read the instructions and apply the technique for you. *Be sure to avoid all direct contact with the joints.*

Massage can be used in conjunction with any alternative therapy, and is often combined with acupressure, aromatherapy, and chiropractic.

Precautions: Do not massage areas of varicose veins or inflammation and swelling due to injury.

To Relieve Muscle Tension

First, apply long, gliding strokes to the area. Then, with the palm of your hand, rub six-inch circles in a counterclockwise direction on the skin. You're ready to release tension from the deep muscles. Take large amounts of skin and muscle into your hands, and work it by squeezing, kneading, and rolling. Work your way up the arm, leg, and so on. You'll feel the tissue soften and become more pliable as you release tensions. Finish by lightly brushing the entire area with your fingertips.

MEDITATION (FOR OSTEOARTHRITIS)

Having arthritis may cause a number of anxieties that affect not only our health but our feeling of well-being as well. We may become absorbed in seeking treatment and avoiding possible "triggers," and at the same time may be trying to cater to others in our lives. Meditation is an inner state of calm that provides us an avenue for letting go of our concerns and allowing peace back into our lives. Meditation calms us and allows us to regain our emotional footing again so that we can calmly face the challenges of each day. Try the practice meditation (see "Meditation," Chapter Three) twice daily to relax.

Meditation can be combined with virtually any natural therapy.

NUTRITIONAL THERAPY (FOR OSTEOARTHRITIS)

In the naturopathic view, arthritis is one of several diseases that are caused by an immune-system reaction as a result of either an allergic reaction to food or eating under stress.

While under stress, the body sends blood to the extremities to prepare for dramatic physical feats, called the "fight or flight" response. Without proper blood flow to the stomach and intestine, these organs cannot digest food properly. Instead of breaking down food into tiny particles, the intestine releases large bits of food into the bloodstream. Before these oversized nutrients can be taken in by organs and tissues, they are attacked by the immune system, which does not recognize them as nutrients due to their large size.

In the second scenario, if food particles are allergens, or substances to which the body is allergic, the immune system will also attack them. In either case, the immune system develops special cells to launch these attacks, and the nutrients become lodged in the joints, causing irritation instead of supplying the tissues as they should.

In order to attack the irritants—the food particles lodged in the joints—the immune system sends more of its cells, but instead of attacking the food particles, the cells malfunction and attack the joints themselves. These immune system attacks throw the body further out of balance and can perpetuate arthritis.

Thus, the treatment for such a problem is to remove the irritant foods from the diet or promote better digestion by chewing food thoroughly and eating only while relaxed. If you are under age sixty-five, going on a five-day partial fast of eating only a well-cooked mixture of equal parts of green beans, zucchini, and okra, which has been liquified in a blender, will allow the digestive tract to heal itself and the immune system to rebalance itself. If allergens are suspected, they can be singularly reintroduced back into the body to test for a reaction, then eliminated from the diet if symptoms reappear.

Another nutritional approach to arthritis involves consuming foods that can benefit the joints. Essential fatty acids such as linoleic acid can replace fatty substances in the synovial fluid that are believed to be lost during disease. Fat lubricates the joints, keeping their surfaces apart so that the cartilage-covered bone ends are protected and can move smoothly. Thus, eating foods containing this oil or taking supplements can help to restore joint lubrication. Vitamin A helps to prevent accumulation of toxic materials in the joints that can contribute to irritation, so ensuring adequate amounts of this nutrient can be helpful. In fact, a vitamin A deficiency can lead to the inadequate production of synovial fluid. Consuming foods that contain adequate amounts of vitamin E, which protects against the destruction of essential fatty acids that lubricate the joints, is also important. Vitamin E and vitamin C are both antioxidants that protect against free radicals, harmful substances that cruise the body, destroy cells, and can contribute to joint pain and irritation. Thus, consuming foods that contain vitamin C is also important.

Because osteoarthritis becomes much more prevalent after menopause, some practitioners believe that it may be partially caused by decline of the hormone estrogen. Therefore, taking nutrients believed to promote estrogen production can be helpful in maximizing the small amounts of the hormone available after the ovaries stop its production. Taking tablets of bee pollen, which contains all twenty-two amino acids, can help to stimulate estrogen production. Bee pollen is available in health-food stores. Similarly, eating unrefined whole grains is believed to promote estrogen production.

Consuming foods with adequate amounts of calcium and phosphorus, which are responsible for laying down and healing bone, may also be effective. Of course, magnesium levels also need to be supplemented. Calcium, magnesium, and phosphorus are all macro minerals, nutrients that are utilized interdependently by the body, so proper ratios must be maintained to avoid deficiency of any of these minerals. Most people with arthritis think that they may be consuming too much calcium when they learn that calcification, or the deposition of calcium, has taken place in the joints. On the contrary, calcification is usually caused by the body's inability to *absorb* calcium, usually as a result of eating excessive amounts of foods containing phosphorus. Thus, cutting back on these foods, which include meat, soda, and processed foods, can be helpful.

A naturally occurring substance called proteoglycans, found in the joints of the body, has also been shown to inhibit the calcification process and minimize irritation. Supplements of this substance, which is made up of 10 percent protein and 90 percent carbohydrates, have been very successful in treating osteoarthritis in Europe.

Also, ensuring adequate amounts of bioflavonoids, which are essential for the production of collagen, a major component of cartilage found in the joints, can enhance cartilage production.

For a list of natural food sources containing these nutrients, see "Nutritional Therapy," Chapter Three.

Glossary

amenorrhea: the abnormal absence of menstruation.

Candida albicans: the most common yeast infection, which can be systemic or just affect the vagina.

cartilage: gristle or smooth, tough tissue that covers the moving surfaces of joints.

cesarean section: surgical delivery of the fetus through the abdominal wall.

collagen: protein that supports bone, cartilage, skin, and connective tissue.

colostrum: this precedes milk in the breast; it is present as early as the second month of pregnancy.

corpus luteum: a small gland found in the ovary that produces progesterone after ovulation. If fertilization occurs, the gland makes the hormones necessary to support the embryo in the first trimester.

corticosteroids: drugs sometimes used to treat asthma or arthritis. Their actions are similar to adrenal hormones.

cyst: a benign, fluid-filled or semisolid lump or sac in any body tissue.

D & C: dilation and curettage. A procedure in which the lining of the uterus (endometrium) and cervix are scraped and examined.

diuretic: a substance that causes the kidney to increase urine production, removing water (and potassium, salt, and iodine) from the body.

dysmenorrhea: abnormally painful or difficult menstrual period.

dysplasia: development of abnormal cells.

edema: swelling as a result of fluid retention.

follicle: a small sac in the ovary containing the developing egg and lined with special cells that produce estrogen and progesterone. After ovulation, the follicle becomes the corpus luteum.

follicle-stimulating hormone (FSH): a hormone produced by the pituitary gland, which, with luteinizing hormone, stimulates the ovary to mature a follicle for ovulation.

hernia: abnormal protrusion of a structure or organ through an opening.

high-density lipoprotein (HDL): a small, dense lipoprotein that sweeps cholesterol from the blood and carries to the liver for excretion.

hyperplasia: excessive growth of normal, not cancerous, cells.

hysterectomy: surgical removal of the uterus. A total hysterectomy includes the ovaries, cervix, and fallopian tubes. A subtotal hysterectomy involves the uterus but not the cervix.

luteinizing hormone (LH): a hormone secreted by the pituitary gland during the menstrual cycle, which is necessary for maturation of an ovarian follicle and release of an egg.

menarche: the onset of the menstrual cycle during puberty.

myomectomy: the surgical removal of a fibroid lump or lumps.

neoplasia: abnormal new growth that can be either malignant or benign.

nulliparity: having never given birth to a live baby.

obesity: being more than 20 percent above desired weight when taking into consideration height, age, sex, bone structure, and muscularity.

oophorectomy: surgical removal of the ovaries.

pelvis: the strong girdle of bone that gives support to the lower part of the body. It consists of the five lowest spinal vertebrae and two hip bones.

perineum: the anatomical area separating the vagina and the rectum.

pica: the craving and ingestion of unusual substances such as clay, baking soda, or earth, often as a result of iron deficiency.

pituitary gland: a gland that secretes hormones and is located at the base of the brain.

placenta: the organ that develops during the third month of pregnancy to channel nutrients and oxygen to the fetus and carry away waste products.

prostaglandins: a group of hormonelike substances that have a wide range of effects on the body that may be good or bad, including regulation of blood pressure, promotion of inflammation, and stimulation of uterine contractions during childbirth.

retrograde menstruation: the backward flow of menstruation through the fallopian tubes and into the pelvic cavity.

toxemia: a condition involving swelling, high blood pressure, and protein in the urine. Also called *preeclampsia* when it appears during the last trimester of pregnancy.

trichomonas: a very irritating vaginal infection that has no serious consequence.

ultrasound: sound waves at a high-pitched frequency, too loud to be heard by humans, that can penetrate human tissue without risk of radiation. Uses include diagnosis during pregnancy and heat therapy for rehabilitation.

vaginal atrophy: a drying and thinning of vaginal tissues.

Natural Medicine Resources

American Association of Acupuncture and Oriental
   Medicine
4101 Lake Boone Trail, Suite 201
Raleigh, NC 27607-6528
(919) 965-7546

American Association of Naturopathic Physicians
P.O. Box 2579
Kirkland, WA 98083-2579
(206) 827-6035

American Association of Orthomolecular Medicine
900 North Federal Highway
Suite 330
Boca Raton, FL 33432
(407) 276-6167

American Chiropractic Association
1701 Clarendon Boulevard
Arlington, VA 22209
(703) 276-8800

American Foundation for Alternative Health Care, Research
   and Development
25 Landfield Avenue
Monticello, NY 12701
(914) 794-8181

American Holistic Nurses Association
4101 Lake Boone Trail, Suite 201
Raleigh, NC 27607
(919) 787-5146

American Holistic Medical Association
2727 Fairview Avenue East
Suite B
Seattle, WA 98102
(206) 322-6842

American Massage Therapy Association
National Information Office
1130 West North Shore Avenue
Chicago, IL 60626
(312) 761-2682

Boston Women's Health Book Collective
465 Mt. Auburn
Watertown, MA 02172
(617) 924-1271

Caesarean Prevention Movement
P.O. Box 152, University Station
Syracuse, NY 10012
(315) 424-1942

Center for Medical Consumers
237 Thompson Street
New York, NY 10012
(212) 674-7105

Coalition for the Medical Rights of Women
1638B Haight Street
San Francisco, CA 94117
(425) 621-8030

Concern for Health Options, Information, Care, and
    Education (CHOICE)
1501 Cherry Street
Philadelphia, PA 19102
(215) 567-2904

Endometriosis Association
U.S.—Canada Headquarters
P.O. Box 92187
Milwaukee, WI 53202
(414) 355-2200

Feminist Action Alliance, Inc.
1300 Spring Street NW
Atlanta, GA 30309
(408) 872-7544

Health Evaluation and Referral Service (HERS)
1954 W. Irving Park Road
Chicago, IL 60613
(312) 248-0166

Human Nutrition Center
6303 Ivy Lane
Greenbelt, MD 20770
(301) 344-2340

International Academy of Nutrition and Preventive
    Medicine
P.O. Box 5832
Lincoln, NE 68505
(402) 467-2716

International Association for Parents and Professionals
    for Safe Alternatives in Childbirth
Route 1, Box 646
Marble Hill, MO 63764
(314) 238-2010

International Childbirth Education Association
P.O. Box 20848
Minneapolis, MN 55420
(612) 854-8660

International Institute of Reflexology
P.O. Box 12462
St. Petersburg, FL 33733
(813) 343-4811

Integral Yoga Institute
227 West 13th Street
New York, NY 10011
(212) 929-0586

National Association for Holistic Aromatherapy
P.O. Box 17622
Boulder, CO 80308
(303) 258-3791

National Accreditation Commission for Schools and
   Colleges of Acupuncture and Oriental Medicine
8403 Colesville Road, Suite 370
Silver Spring, MD 20919
(301) 608-9680

National Center for Homeopathy
801 North Fairfax, Suite 306
Alexandria, VA 22314
(703) 548-7790

National Commission for the Certification of Acupuncturists
1424 16 Street NW, Suite 501
Washington, DC 20036
(202) 232-1401

National Foundation for Women's Health
342 W 22nd Street
New York, NY 10011
(212) 924-6863

National Women's Health Network
2025 I Street NW, Suite 105
Washington, DC 20006
(202) 233-6886

National Women's Health Organization
110 East 59th Street
New York, NY 10022
(212) 355-5420

Waterbirth International
P.O. Box 5554
Santa Barbara, CA 93150
(800) 565-3980

Women's Action Alliance, Inc.
370 Lexington Avenue
New York, NY 10017
(212) 532-8330

Women's Occupational Health Resource Center
School of Public Health
Columbia University
60 Haven Avenue
New York, NY 10017
(212) 781-5719

Herb Sources

Annandale Apothecary
7023 Little River Turnpike
Annandale, VA 22003

Boerick and Tafel, Inc.
1011 Arch Street
Philadelphia, PA 19107
or
2381 Circadian Way
Santa Rosa, CA 95407

Boiron-Borneman, Inc.
6 Campus Blvd.
Bldg. A
Newtown Square, PA 19073

Ehrhart and Karl
17 North Wabash Avenue
Chicago, IL 60602

Herbarium
264 Exchange Street
Chicopee, MA 01013

Horton and Converse
621 West Pico Blvd.
Los Angeles, CA 90015

Humphreys Pharmacal Company
63 Meadow Road
Rutherford, NJ 07070

Keihl Pharmacy, Inc.
109 Third Avenue
New York, NY 10003

Luyties Pharmacal Company
4200 Laclede Avenue
St. Louis, MO 63108

Mylans Homeopathic Pharmacy
222 O'Farrell Street
San Francisco, CA 94102

Running Fox Farm (flower essences)
74 Thrashing Hill Road
Worthington, MA 01098
(413) 238-4291

Santa Monica Drug
1513 Fourth Street
Santa Monica, CA 90401

Standard Homeopathic Company
204–210 West 131 Street
Los Angeles, CA 90061

Washington Homeopathic Pharmacy
4914 Delray Avenue
Bethesda, MD 20814

Weleda, Inc.
841 South Main Street
Spring Valley, NY 10977

Acupressure Points

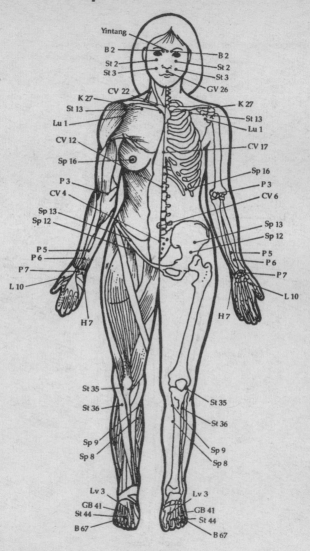

Front View

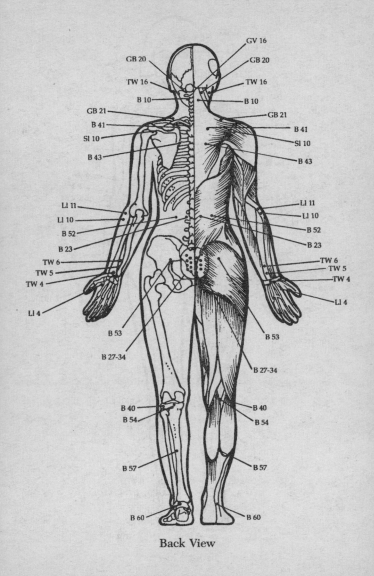

Back View

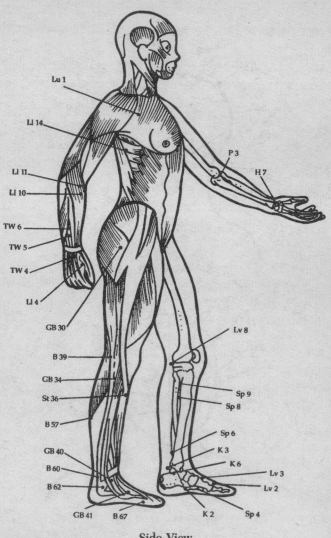

Side View

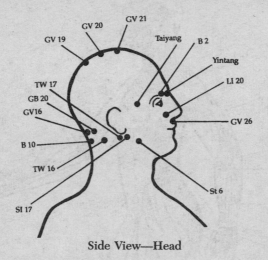

Side View—Head

GV 19 · GV 20 · GV 21 · Taiyang · B 2 · Yintang · LI 20 · GV 26 · TW 17 · GB 20 · GV 16 · B 10 · TW 16 · SI 17 · St 6

Front View—Head

Yintang · B 2 · St 2 · LI 20 · St 3 · B 2 · St 2 · LI 20 · St 3 · GV 26

The Natural Medicine Collective

BIOGRAPHIES

Dr. William Bergman *(Homeopathy)*

William Bergman holds an M.D. degree from Columbia University and has completed postgraduate physicians' programs sponsored by the National Center for Homeopathy, the International Foundation for Homeopathy, and the United States Homeopathic Association. He is the medical director of Hahnemann Health Associates, one of the most comprehensive homeopathic medical and educational facilities in New York. Dr. Bergman also serves as the president of the World Medical Health Foundation, Inc., an organization researching the cause, treatment, and prevention of disease.

Brian Clement *(Nutrition)*

Brian Clement is the director of the Hippocrates Institute, the first progressive health center in this country. A founding director of the Coalition of Holistic Health, he has served as director at health centers in Denmark and Greece and has consulted at holistic clinics throughout the world. With over twenty years of international leadership experience in the field of alternative health care, he has appeared on numerous radio and television shows and has conducted hundreds of workshops and seminars on natural medicine.

Dr. Brian Fradet *(Chiropractic, Panel Coordinator)*

Brian Fradet holds a doctorate of chiropractic from the prestigious New York Chiropractic College and has completed postgraduate research in neurology at the New York University Medical Center. He is a longstanding member of the American Chiropractic Association, the Foundation for Chiropractic Education and Research, the Parker Chiropractic Research Foundation, the New York State Chiropractic Association, and the Chiropractic Federated Society of New York. He is the founder of the Fradet Pain Clinic in New York.

Elaine Retholtz, L.Ac. *(Acupuncture)*

Elaine Retholtz is a licensed acupuncturist and a diplomate of the National Commission for the Certification of Acupuncturists. She is a graduate of the Tri-State Institute of Traditional Chinese Acupuncture. She holds a master's degree in nutritional sciences from the University of Wisconsin—Madison. She maintains a private practice in New York specializing in acupuncture. She is the supervising acupuncturist for Crossroads: An Alternative for Women Offenders—A Project of the Center for Community Alternatives (formerly National Center on Institutions and Alternatives/Northeast).

Dr. James Lawrence Thomas *(Psychology)*

James Lawrence Thomas is a licensed psychologist and neuropsychologist with postdoctoral certificates in cognitive, relationship, group, and grief therapy. He is on the faculty of the New York University Medical Center and has served as the consulting neuropsychologist to Mt. Sinai Medical Center's Department of Neurology. He holds degrees from Yale, the University of California, Berkeley, and City University of

New York. Dr. Thomas maintains a private practice in New York.

Dr. Maurice H. Werness, Jr. *(Naturopathy)*

Maurice H. Werness, Jr., received a doctoral degree from the Bastyr College of Naturopathic Medicine. He is the medical director of Healingheart Healthcare, one of the West Coast's most prominent facilities for holistic care. He is also the director of development at the Institute for Naturopathic Medicine. A former tennis professional, Dr. Werness is the founder and director of True Tennis, an organization that teaches tennis and health education to physically and emotionally challenged people.

Rebecca Papas is a freelance health writer who has written numerous articles on women's health topics for newspapers and magazines. She has served as a writer and editor for the prestigious Joslin Diabetic Center quarterly, *Joslin Magazine*. She lives in New York City.

Index